Critical Acclaim for the First Edition

"**The Validation Breakthrough** will inform and reassure families involved in the demanding and stressful task of caring for elderly people with dementia. The book is indeed timely."

Maggie Kuhn
Founder, Gray Panthers

"For those struggling with the obsolete practices of reality orientation, Naomi Feil's latest book unlocks the doors of communicating positively with the person with Alzheimer's disease. Her **Validation Breakthrough** is a win-win approach, allowing caregivers to truly be 'givers of care' in providing compassionate care while improving the quality of care and life of the person with Alzheimer's disease. Naomi has revived, for the long-term care industry, the medical adage 'do no harm.'"

Mary Lucero, B.S.H., N.H.A.
President, Geriatric Resources, Inc.

"Naomi Feil presents an artful, sensitive, and caring intervention approach to working with confused and disoriented older adults. The case studies and examples are rich with insight and provide clear examples of techniques that may be used. The approach is empowering to older adults and to their caregivers."

Harvey L. Sterns, Ph.D.
Director
Institute for Life-Span Development and Gerontology
The University of Akron

"Feil is one of the very few people in the field who has dealt with the emotional aspects of advanced Alzheimer's disease. Her new book is written with humor, sensitivity, respect, and genuine sympathy. It is an important addition to the literature."

Ruth Tappen, Ed.D., R.N.
Professor of Nursing
Florida Atlantic University

"The Validation Breakthrough demonstrates in a powerful way how Validation therapy actually works. It is must reading for anyone who works with the elderly. The communication tools outlined will greatly reduce the frustration and burnout often experienced by the caregiver. This book will leave you inspired!"

Scott Averill, J.D., N.H.A.
Administrator
Colonial Manor of Lansing, Kansas
Beverly Enterprises

"Validation therapy is a way to create person-to-person connections that can light up the lives of elderly individuals mistakenly thought to be beyond reach. And, mysteriously and wonderfully, as I've seen Validation working, I've discovered that applying this method seems to kindle within the person using it a renewed sense of meaning, an affirmation of self that is its own best reward."

Paula McClain Mixson, C.S.W.
Board member (1988–1992)
National Gray Panthers

The
Validation
Breakthrough

Publisher's note: The subtitle of this book, *Simple Techniques for Communicating with People with "Alzheimer's-Type Dementia,"* may be confusing to some readers. As used here, the term *Alzheimer's-type dementia* is intended to include people in their late 70s or older who have lost some recent memory; who have some sensory impairment; and who have been *diagnosed* as having senile dementia of the Alzheimer's type, dementia, or Alzheimer's disease. Some people diagnosed as having Alzheimer's disease may not actually have this condition. A definitive diagnosis of Alzheimer's disease is possible only on autopsy, when the brain of the deceased person is inspected for plaques and tangles. Dementia or disorientation is often caused by a multitude of factors other than Alzheimer's disease, including some loss of memory, eyesight, hearing, work, family, and friends.

The Validation Breakthrough

Simple Techniques for Communicating with People with "Alzheimer's-Type Dementia"

Second Edition

by

Naomi Feil, M.S.W., A.C.S.W.
Executive Director
Validation Training Institute
Cleveland, Ohio

Revised by
Vicki de Klerk-Rubin

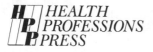
HEALTH
PROFESSIONS
PRESS

Baltimore • London • Winnipeg • Sydney

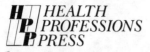

HEALTH PROFESSIONS PRESS

Health Professions Press, Inc.
Post Office Box 10624
Baltimore, Maryland 21285-0624
www.healthpropress.com

Typeset by TechBooks, York, Pennsylvania.
Manufactured in the United States of America by
Versa Press, East Peoria, Illinois.

Permission to reprint the photographs on the following pages is
gratefully acknowledged:
Pages 67 and 235: Steven R. Jones and Elizabeth C. Zimmerman
Page 84: Joy Goodwin and Agnes Maske
Page 119: Rita Altman and Ethel Warner
Page 148: Ann Gurnett and Pam Amos
Page 171: Joy Goodwin and Alice Dalton
Page 223: Rita Altman, Theresa Benkovic, and Ethel Warner
Page 255: Shirley Orr, Margaret McLeay, Graham Weil, and
Fred Skinner
Photograph on page xiii by Clifford Norton Studio
Photographs on pages 13, 43, 62, 77, and 93 by Edward R. Feil

Library of Congress Cataloging-in-Publication Data

Feil, Naomi.
    The validation breakthrough: simple techniques for
    communicating with people with Alzheimer's-type dementia / by
    Naomi Feil.—2nd ed.
    p.   cm.
    Includes bibliographical references and index.
    ISBN 1-878812-81-5
    1. Alzheimer's disease—Patients—Care. 2. Senile
    dementia—Patients—Care. 3. Validation therapy. I. Title.
RC523 .F454   2002
616.8'3106—dc21   2001051784

British Library Cataloguing in Publication data are available from the
British Library.

Contents

About the Author

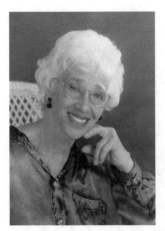

Naomi Feil, M.S.W., A.C.S.W., is the Executive Director of the Validation Training Institute, in Cleveland, Ohio. She is the creator of Validation, currently recognized throughout the world as a state-of-the-art therapy for older people diagnosed as having Alzheimer's dementia or related disorders.

Ms. Feil earned her master's of social work from Columbia University and studied at the New School for Social Research, Case Western Reserve University, and the University of Michigan. In 1963, she became dissatisfied with traditional therapies for older people with dementia and began to develop her own methods for helping older people cope with the disorientation that is sometimes part of the aging process.

In addition to her earlier book on Validation, Ms. Feil has published numerous journal articles and has produced nine award-winning films on Validation. The first edition of *The Validation Breakthrough: Simple Techniques for Communicating with People with "Alzheimer's-Type Dementia"* has sold 40,000 copies. She is internationally recognized for her work with older people and is one of the most sought-after trainers in the field. More than 30,000 facilities in the United States of America, Canada, Europe, and Australia have adopted Validation, and nearly 90,000 professional and family caregivers have attended her workshops in North America, Australia, and Europe. There are 16 Validation centers that teach Validation certification courses in 11 countries. In Switzerland, every agency that serves older people uses Validation.

Vicki de Klerk-Rubin is the European manager of the Validation Training Institute, a certified Validation trainer, and the co-author of the 1992 revision of *Validation: The Feil Method.* Ms. de Klerk-Rubin holds a bachelor of fine arts from Boston University and a master of business administration from Fordham University and is a Dutch-trained registered nurse. Ms. de Klerk-Rubin has given Validation workshops, lectures, and training programs in Austria, Belgium, England, Finland, France, Germany, the Netherlands, Sweden, Italy, and the United States of America. She also has worked in numerous nursing facilities in Amsterdam, leading Validation groups and training staff.

I dedicate this book to my editor and friend, Lita Kohn, without whom it would never have been written. Her guidance, enthusiasm, and honest search for what makes life meaningful have helped me look forward to my old-old age.

Foreword

Country Meadows Retirement Communities, founded in 1983, was one of the first assisted living providers to design a special program of compassionate care for people living with Alzheimer's disease and related dementias. Our philosophy has always been to help our residents build on their remaining strengths, while minimizing their limitations.

When I first learned of the work of Naomi Feil in 1997, I realized that here is someone offering a method that takes the human being into account, recognizing the older disoriented person's inner wisdom.

We invited Naomi to talk to our co-workers about Validation. I was tremendously impressed when I saw her put the Validation method into practice with one of our residents. Within a matter of minutes, she was able to restore dignity and reduce the anxiety of an agitated resident. With empathetic listening, using Validation techniques, she entered the resident's inner world. The Validation method built trust. The resident was no longer afraid and alone.

I knew that it would be important for our co-workers, who routinely work with our confused residents, to have an opportunity to learn and be able to implement the Validation method. In 1999, Country Meadows' in-house training institute, the George M. Leader Institute, became the first Authorized Validation Organization (AVO) in the United States of America. Since then, several hundred co-workers have received orientation in the Validation method, including 13 who have completed higher level certification in Group Validation.

The most sincere stories of the impact of Validation come from the workers who have been able to successfully implement their Validation skills with residents. We are rewarded by the accolades our co-workers have received from family members who are seeing their mothers and fathers become more social and experience fewer episodes of emotional outbursts. Repeatedly, co-workers enthusiastically report that residents are finally being understood because of the Validation principles they are using. Perhaps, more important, one of the greatest benefits of Validation is the ability to reduce anxiety without the use of psychotropic drugs.

You have in your hands a book with vivid examples and techniques that help restore dignity to the older confused person, reduce frustration, and give joy to the caregiver.

I am tremendously grateful to Naomi Feil and her daughter, Vicki de Klerk-Rubin, for their tireless efforts to develop and promote the idea that there is a reason behind some of the unusual, and oftentimes disruptive, behaviors common with those who are diagnosed with an Alzheimer's-related dementia.

This book is for anyone who is interested in developing more meaningful interactions with confused seniors.

George M. Leader
Founder and Chairman Emeritus
Country Meadows Retirement Communities
Hershey, Pennsylvania

Authorized Validation Organizations

Australia
Alan Johns
Validation Therapy
   Training and Resource
   Centre
Post Office Box 939
   Eltham
Victoria 3095, Australia
Telephone/fax: (61) (3) 9888
   4968

Austria
Validation Training Center
   at Ausbildungszentrum
   des Wiener Roten
   Kreuzes
Franzosengraben 8
A-1030 Vienna, Austria
Telephone: (43) (1) 795
   806300
Fax: (43) (1) 795 809610

Belgium
Didier Barbieux
Rhapsodie
Chaussée de Waterloo 788
1180 Brussels
Belgium
Telephone: (32) (2) 372 2351
Fax: (32) (2) 372 2332

Denmark
Kirsten Sejerøe-Szatkowski
The Danish Validation
   Association
Højlundvej 6, Voervadsbro
8660 Skanderborg
Denmark
Telephone: (45) (75) 78 21
   74
Fax: (45) (75) 78 21 52

Finland
Satu Sipola
Tampere City Mission
Aleksanterinkatu 23 D
33100 Tampere, Finland
Telephone: (358) (3) 212
   0017
Fax: (358) (3) 212 2878

France
Association pour la
   promotion de
   la Validation Therapy,
   secretariat
26, rue de la Carrièra
68800 Thann, France
Telephone: (33) (3) 893
   71163
Fax: (33) (3) 893 71523

Germany
Saarland, Rheinland-Pfalz
Hessen, Thuringen:
Fachbereich Validation
Landesverein für Innere
  Mission in der Pfalz
Dr. Kaufmann Strasse 2
67098 Bad Dürkheim
Telephone: 06322/ 607 230
Fax: 06322/ 607 103

Baden Württemberg,
  Bayern,
Nordrhein-Westfalen:
Wolfgang Hahl
Deutsches Rotes Kreuz
Kreisverband Mannheim
Postfach 120465
68055 Mannheim
Telephone: 0621/ 833 7040
Fax: 0621/ 833 7049

Niedersachsen,
  Sachsen-Anhalt,
Brandenburg,
  Mecklenburg-
  Vorpommern, Schleswig
Holstein:
Insitut für Angewandte
Gerontologie
Haubachstrasse 8
10585 Berlin, Germany
Telephone: (49) (30) 341
  5034
Fax: (49) (30) 341 6068

The Netherlands
Stichting Validation
Anklaarseweg 91
7316 MC Apeldoorn,
  Netherlands
Telephone: (31) (55) 578
  9339
Fax: (31) (55) 576 1410

Sweden
Kristina Telerud
Ersta diakonisällskap
Erstagatan 1
11691 Stockholm, Sweden
Telephone: (46) (8) 714
  6689, 714 6217
Fax: (46) (8) 714 6673

Switzerland
Tertianum ZfP
Kronenhof
CH-8267 Berlingen TG
Switzerland
Telephone: (41) (52) 762
  5757
Fax: (41) (52) 762 5770

United States of America
Jana Stoddard
Validation Training Center
  at George M. Leader
  Institute
830 Cherry Drive
Hershey, Pennsylvania
  17033 USA

Telephone: (01) (717) 533
2474

Fax: (01) (717) 533 6202

Validation Training Center
at Virginia
Commonwealth
University
1101 East Marshal Street
Post Office Box 980568
Richmond, Virginia 23298
Telephone: (01) (804) 828
5188

**Validation Training
Institute, Incorporated**
21987 Byron Road
Cleveland, Ohio 44122

Telephone: (01) (216) 651
0357

Fax: (01) (216) 751 6434

E-mail: naomifeil@aol.com

**Validation Training
Institute European
Manager**
Vicki de Klerk-Rubin
Wohllebengasse 7/9
1040 Vienna, Austria
Telephone: (43) (1) 503
8434
Fax: (43) (1) 503 843420
E-mail:
penvdek@attglobal.net

Introduction

Florence Trew
1872–1963: "I died"

I write this book for Florence Trew, a resident of a nursing home, and for the millions of very old people like her. I was 8 and she was 68 in December 1940 when we first met.

I grew up in a Home for the Aged. You had to be 65 or older to get into The Home. I got in because my father, a psychologist, was the administrator. My mother, the first master's degree social worker to work in a Home for the Aged, established the Social Service Department in 1943.

Mrs. Trew was my best friend in The Home. I was never allowed to call her by her first name. She was always Mrs. Trew. She was tall and well-built, with a fine, longish thin nose on which she perched her bifocal lorgnette. Mrs. Trew would often shake her head up and down to make a point, her glasses bobbing dangerously, dancing at the very tip of her nose. Mrs. Trew read to me. I loved her low, clear, resonant voice. Her voice soothed me. Her voice trembled only once, when she read me a page in her diary.

She had found me sobbing on the cracked pavement leading to The Home. My feet were tangled in roller skate straps. Mrs. Trew plunked herself beside me to catch every word. I explained that my mother had given my brother and me new roller skates. My brother's skates were elegantly etched with the word *Rollfast*. My skates, in much smaller letters, said *Skinner*. I told Mrs. Trew that my mother loved my brother better. My skates were much skinnier than my brother's, which is why he sailed gracefully far ahead, leaving me clunking, an awkward robot, far behind.

Mrs. Trew understood these inequities. To heal my hurt, she produced her diary, which she always carried in her big black shiny purse. Mrs. Trew found the page she wanted with her fingers, without looking. She touched the paper and froze. She squeezed her eyes shut. Suddenly, her eyes flared wide open, two blue question marks. We stared at each other, silently sharing misery.

Mrs. Trew began to read to me from her diary. Her sweet lyrical voice changed to a dull, flat, lifeless monotone. The words on the page spoke themselves without her soul.

June 10, 1891

Dear Diary:

My mother hasn't changed. She embarrassed me again today, just like she did in Miss Nelson's third-grade class- room. Remember, Diary? It was Tuesday, Parent–Teacher Night. She was talking to Miss Nelson just before the bell rang. My mother pointed her finger at me while she was talking, making everybody look at me. I scrunched myself down and willed myself to vanish. She whispered in a very loud voice, "Florence can't let go of that ugly wooden rab- bit. That's why she has no friends." She bent down close to Sally Quinn in the first row. "Honey, would you be friends with someone who drags a wooden rabbit around wherever she goes? No! You wouldn't!" Sally Quinn gig- gled. My mother was satisfied. The whole class giggled. My mother made her point and turned back to Miss Nelson. "I'm worried about Florence. I don't want her lugging that creaky rabbit around all her life." My mother didn't even bother to whisper. She moved toward me un- til she towered over me, holding out her hand for Creaky. "Creaky is mine," I said. I loved Creaky so much that I stuttered. I held his string tighter, hiding him under my desk. Daddy had made him for my third birthday, just before he left us for good.

> *Creaky's white pointed ears were smooth as velvet.*
> *Touching them made me feel peaceful, almost as if Daddy*
> *were with me. Daddy tied the string around Creaky's neck*
> *so that I could pull him behind me. Creaky's joints made a*
> *wonderful crackling sound when I pulled. I always knew*
> *he was there. My mother grabbed Creaky so hard that*
> *his hind leg snapped off. She marched up front and threw*
> *Creaky into Miss Nelson's steel wastebasket. Creaky made*
> *a hollow sound as he hit the bottom. I ran up to save him.*
> *Miss Nelson took the wastebasket with Creaky away.*

Mrs. Trew closed her diary and her eyes. I put my hand in hers. "What happened then?" I whispered.

"I died," she answered.

I said goodbye to my friend Mrs. Trew in 1950. She stayed in The Home, and I went to New York City to study psychology and social work at Columbia University. In 1956, I began working with older people in community centers in New York. In 1963, I returned to Cleveland to do postgraduate studies, to teach, and to work with the disoriented residents at The Home where I grew up.

The summer of 1963 was hot and humid. The windows were open in the day room of the Special Service Wing for Wandering and Disoriented Residents of The Home. "Help me! Help me!" Pleading voices drifted everywhere. No one turned to look. No one listened. The day room was bright, lit by the sun spotlighting rows of heads slumped in geri-chairs. The bodies were tied with white restraints. A few sat straight up, staring bleakly into space.

I was drawn to a white shapeless form in a chair. It was an emaciated woman with paper-thin arms laced with blue veins. Like a vise, the massive chair, with its over-sized back and flat wooden tray in the front, trapped the tiny old woman. Mechanically, she pounded the metallic tray imprisoning her. "Cree. Cree. Cree," her low scratchy voice belched. The sound was eerie. Her hands caressed an invisible object, stroking something only she could see. Her head wobbled, cradled by bony shoulders. Loose strands of thin hair drifted into her blue eyes. She wore a house-dress sprinkled with faded pink rosebuds, washed too many times, and torn terry cloth slippers. She grabbed my wrist and held it tight. I looked at her long fingers, the nails brittle, her forearm splotched with liver spots. Bulging purple veins branched from each knuckle to her tiny wrist. I saw her name band.

"Florence Trew." Could this be the same Florence Trew? I saw Mrs. Trew in my mind's eye. Twenty years earlier she had been 65 years old. When we were last together, we had sung "I've Been Workin' on the Railroad!" together. Residents had shuffled by, shaking their heads in disapproval. Later, we had walked 7 miles to the movie theater on Euclid Heights Boulevard. We got in free because we lived in The Home. We shared a bag of popcorn and gaped at Flash Gordon. We were a team. Together, we had earned 30 cents a day picking spongy red rubber from worn-out tires to benefit the war effort. The two of us had won the Red Rubber Pickers Award. Mrs. Trew had hung the medal on her door.

My memory stuck in my throat as I bent down to meet her eyes. "Remember our medal, Mrs. Trew? Remember the war effort? Remember the Red Rubber Pickers?" She heard. She looked straight into my eyes, locking them. She whispered my nickname, "Mimi. Mimi, get me out of this chair."

"You can't untie her," the nursing assistant warned me. "She fell three times last week trying to get away. If you untie her and she falls again, you are responsible."

"What happened?" I whispered to Mrs. Trew, bending very close.

"They threw him away. Make them give him back, Mimi. Please." Mrs. Trew's voice held the same soft ring of long ago. Her blue eyes were clear. Her hands holding mine were strong.

"Who?" I asked. "Mrs. Trew, who did they take away from you?"

"Creaky. She threw him in the wastebasket." Mrs. Trew pointed to the nurse.

"That's the nurse, Mrs. Trew, not your mother."

Mrs. Trew shook her head, disappointed in me. She turned away, tuning me out to stare into space, moaning softly, "Cree. Cree. Cree."

I persisted. "Mrs. Trew, did you have a stroke?" I wondered about her recent memory. She stared at me, speechless. Her lips formed words but no sound. She sat limp, resigned, conforming her body to the restraints. She sighed, "I'm dead."

I argued. "Mrs. Trew, you can't be dead. You are talking to me!"

"Honey, you are hearing things," Mrs. Trew said sadly.

"Do you want to die, Mrs. Trew?" I asked softly.

"Yes." Her answer was sharp and clear. "Creaky and I are rubbish. Red rubber rubbish. Rub. Rub. Rub a dub dub. Throw us in the trash can!"

Mrs. Trew's voice rose suddenly to a shriek, piercing the day room. She hurled the imaginary object across the floor.

"Shut up, lady!" A hoarse male voice bounced back.

"SHUT UP!" A chorus of voices bleated.

Mrs. Trew started to cry, whispering between sobs, "Poor Creaky. She tore your legs. Your white ear is so soft. Get me out of this chair. Help! Help!" Mrs. Trew screamed.

I put my arms around Mrs. Trew.

A hoarse male voice shouted, "She's nuts, lady. You can't help her. Help me! Get these offa' me!" The very old man tugged at his restraints. The strong white fabric would not give an inch. Frustrated, his voice topped Mrs. Trew's. The day room became a chorus of out-of-tune voices. "Help! Get me out of here! Shut up. Son of a bitch! Give 'em all chloroform!"

The nursing assistant gave me a dirty look. Her sharp voice cut through the wails. "You're getting them all worked up. Once they start, you can't stop them." She tightened Mrs. Trew's restraint with a brisk, efficient yank as she spoke. Mrs. Trew swished her foot hard against the nursing assistant's shin. Mrs. Trew hollered, "Give me back Creaky, you bitch! I hate you! All the children in this classroom hate you!"

Controlled, patient, and calm, the nursing assistant moistened her lips with her tongue. She waved her arm at the old figures slumped in geri-chairs. "Please don't upset them, Naomi. You can't help them. I've been working here for 5 years, and I ought to know."

She never looked at Mrs. Trew but grabbed her chair and wheeled her quickly down the long hallway, talking to the chair back. "Sweetie, you shouldn't use those bad words. You know better than that. A bitch," she explained patiently, "is a female dog. I am not a female dog. I am your nurse, and I love you. It's time to go beddy-by. Everything will be just fine, honey." Her voice drifted, honey toned, through the corridor and finally faded.

Mrs. Trew never had a chance to turn her head to look back at me. Mrs. Trew and I never had a chance to say good-bye. She died that night.

I spent the next 30 years working with people like Mrs. Trew. I developed Validation, a way of communicating with them. The very old disoriented people taught me. I learned from their social histories, their families, their nurses, and their friends. I learned by mistakes. I learned that very old disoriented people have an intuitive wisdom, a basic humanity that we all share. Behind their disorientation lies a human knowing. This humanity stretches beyond present time, culture, race, geography, and religion. When present time and place fade, when work goes, when rules no longer matter, when social obligations have lost meaning, a basic humanity shines through.

Nature helps these very old people find their inner wisdom. When their eyes fail and the outside world blurs, very old people look inside. They use their vivid mind's eye to see. People from the past become real. When recent memory goes and time blurs, very old people begin to measure life in terms of memories, not minutes. When the very old lose their speech, similar sounds, rhythms, and early learned movements substitute for words. To survive the present-day losses, the very old restore the past. They find much wisdom in the past.

I write this book for four reasons. First, I write so that sons, daughters, nurses, doctors, neighbors, and friends will learn how to use Validation. They will learn to walk beside the very old person in this final life stage. They will learn empathy. They will learn to listen and talk with the disoriented instead of restraining them or patronizing them or telling them what to do. They will learn to respect them.

Second, I write so that the caregiver will find some pleasure in being with the very old disoriented person. A 50-year-old daughter who understands why her mother packs her bag to see a long-dead husband can relate to her mother. The daughter will learn more about her own parent. A nurse who knows how to touch a slumped, speechless figure can spark a memory of a mother's touch. The old woman's eyes light. Her lips form a word. Her body straightens. The nurse and the old woman sing a familiar lullaby. The old woman does not know the nurse's name, but the old woman loves the nurse. The nurse feels joy in being loved and giving new life to the old woman. The interaction takes 3 minutes.

Third, I write for all of us who will become very old and who want to age successfully. When we gain empathy with the disoriented, we begin to understand the reasons behind their disorientation. We can learn the ingredients for successful aging. We can gain insight into our own hang-ups. We can learn to recognize our own unresolved life tasks. We can work on completing these tasks now—before we reach very old age. We can find a repertoire for coping with losses. If we face scary feelings when we're young, then we won't be stuck with a backpack of dirty laundry when we get to be very old. We need to prepare for old age while our speech, logic, and social controls are intact and we have the capacity to change.

Finally, I write for younger generations who will become caregivers. In 2000, there were 10 million Americans older than 80. We want our caregivers to understand us, not restrain us. If our controls have weakened, if we expose our sores, if our feelings, as well as our bladders, should become incontinent, we do not want to be tranquilized. We do not want to be labeled "senile delinquents." If buried rage surfaces out of sequence—in the final life stage instead of in adolescence—we want empathy.

Mrs. Trew controlled her feelings throughout her life. She buried her anger at her mother. Only after age 80—after she lost physical controls, after she lost her husband, her home, her daughter, her clear vision, her recent memory, and her mobility—did she relive her painful memory. Over and over, in the day room of the nursing home, she yelled at her mother. The nurse was a blur. Mrs. Trew's optic nerve was damaged, but she could focus clearly with her mind's eye. She used the nurse's shadowy form to restore her mother. She transformed the blurry figures in wheelchairs to children sitting behind desks in a third-grade classroom.

Mrs. Trew had entered the Resolution Stage of life. Her final task: to clean the slate before she died. She returned to the past to resolve old hurts. Eight-year-old Florence never shouted, "MOTHER, I DIED THE DAY YOU THREW CREAKY IN THE WASTEBASKET!" She waited 80 years. She waited too long.

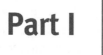

Part I

Alzheimer's-Type Dementia and the Use of Validation

Part I includes nine chapters. In Chapter 1, I describe the normal process of aging and human development and identify the crucial social and psychological needs of the "old-old." In Chapter 2, the concept of Validation is introduced, and I describe the characteristic stages of very old people who enter the final struggle—what I call the Resolution Stage of life— and describe the Validation techniques that can help restore dignity in each stage.

Chapters 3, 4, 5, and 6 present vivid case histories of people in progressive stages of Resolution—Malorientation,

Time Confusion, Repetitive Motion, and Vegetation. All of these chapters describe the physical and psychological characteristics typical of each stage of Resolution and reveal how Validation has helped both the disoriented old-old and the people who have cared for them.

Chapter 7 deals with the special case of early-onset Alzheimer's disease—Alzheimer's dementia that begins before the age of 70. Validation has been much less effective with these people than it has with people who become disoriented in their 80's or 90's. Unlike the old-old disoriented, people with early-onset Alzheimer's disease deteriorate despite Validation. However, caregivers who work with people with early-onset Alzheimer's dementia have found some short-term benefits of Validation, as described in Chapter 7.

Chapter 8 looks at some of the research that has been conducted on the effect of Validation on the disoriented old-old, on the professionals and paraprofessionals who have cared for them, and on the families of disoriented old people. As this chapter shows, positive effects for all three groups have repeatedly been shown.

Finally, Chapter 9 examines the differences between Validation and seven other interventions that are often used with disoriented older adults—reality orientation, behavior modification, psychotherapy, diversion, life review, reminiscence, and remotivation.

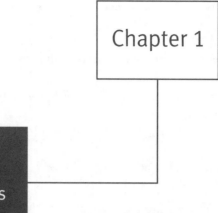

Chapter 1

Aging,
Development,
and Alzheimer's
Disease

HOW I LEARNED: THE CASE OF ISADORE ROSE: "YOU CASTRATED ME WITH WORDS"

Isadore Rose was a tall, bony, good-looking man when we met. He moved with purpose and was oriented to present time and place, but he was not happily oriented. He was *maloriented*. He was loaded with emotional scars from the past, suffering from feelings he had not faced earlier in life. In 1963, I did not know about an individual's final struggle, what I came to call the Resolution Stage of life. I judged Isadore by standards of behavior that apply to old people who are not stuck with unfinished life tasks. I misunderstood him and the many people like him.

In 1963, I found Isadore Rose struggling to tie up loose ends. Before we were even introduced, he whispered to me that his sister, Helen, was saving money by not feeding him enough. His sister amazed me with her compassion for this bitter old man. Together, after his death, Helen and I tried to understand Isadore. We began with his nursing home history.

His final record reflected his sad existence:

Assets: 1 black suit, 3 shirts, 1 pr. pajamas, 1 pr. shorts, 1 Schick razor, 1 pr. shoes

Personal savings: None

Financial arrangement: Monthly veteran's pension

Medical diagnosis: CVA with left herniparesis. Paget's disease of the bone. Osteochondroma right tibia. Bowel surgery 1955 for enteritis. Prostate surgery 1963.

Psychiatric diagnosis: Chronic organic brain syndrome, senile dementia-type

Certificate of death: Isadore Rose died on 1/6/73 at 11:45 A.M. Approximate interval between onset and death: 5 minutes. Immediate cause: respiratory arrest.

Through Helen, I learned about Isadore's earlier life. "He wanted so much to be loved," she told me. Her voice was hollow, the deep circles under her eyes made her face puffy and ghostlike. "To be somebody. Our father never loved him. He punished Isadore by locking him in the attic. In my dreams, even today, I hear Father yell, 'You are no good, Isadore. You'll never amount to anything.' Isadore never yelled back. I never saw him cry."

"You know, Isadore was born at the wrong time. Our parents couldn't afford another child. They had just come to America from Russia, without a penny. Mother hid me under her sewing machine in the factory where she worked. I was 2 years old. When the boss found me, he fired her, and she was pregnant with Isadore." Helen Wallace's words rushed one on top of the other, spinning out her life.

"I know it wasn't Isadore's fault that his wife divorced him. She kept saying that he was impotent. He wanted more than anything to have a child. Isadore was waiting for the day when he could get season baseball tickets for a son. Father never once took Isadore anywhere, not even to a ball game. When Isadore's wife left him, he moved in with us. He helped us pay for our house, but he was never a successful lawyer. When he lost the Ephraim Gross case, his one big case, he gave up. He said the judge didn't like him, so what was the use of trying. He barely earned a living after that. Poor guy! Every day, he walked up the hill to his law office on Buckeye and 116th Street. I don't know what he did there all day. Then he fell. The doctor said he had a bone disease. He tried so hard to keep walking. He fell down our basement steps and said it was my fault. He said I didn't feed him enough. Crazy! On top of that, he wouldn't sign his Social Security checks. He said we would steal them. That's when I called you, almost 11 years ago. My God! I can't believe it's been so long!"

Together, Helen and I reviewed Isadore's sad later life, beginning in 1962, when he had begun attending day care. With the benefit of hindsight, these excerpts from his history struck me as a chronicle of missed opportunities:

3/62: Isadore Rose, age 73, enrolls in day care center. Client is mildly confused, usually continent. Claims his sister is stealing his pension. Staff instructed to use reality orientation with client.

5/62: Client accuses center director of abusing him and locking him in the attic. Appears agitated and swears angrily at staff. Staff assure client that nobody would hurt him. Reality orientation does not seem to be effective with client.

4/63: Client undergoes prostate surgery. Although surgery is successful, he accuses surgeon of castrating him. Seems more confused after surgery, seems to swear at staff more.

5/63: Client seen by psychiatrist, diagnosed with schizophrenia with hallucinations, senile dementia with chronic organic brain syndrome. Behavior modification recommended to deal with unacceptable behaviors. Day care staff instructed to ignore client when he becomes aggressive.

8/63: Behavior modification not working. Client becomes physically abusive when ignored. Day care staff unable to deal with client.

3/69: Client admitted to nursing home. Incontinent most of the time. Client blames incontinence on administrator.

4/69: Social worker sees client, reports failure to connect with him. Client turns head away, scribbles on legal pad—which he carries with him at all time—when social worker tries to provide insight into his behaviors.

10/70: Client refuses to talk, keeps eyes shut. Handwriting shows much deterioration.

3/71: Client restrained in wheelchair during waking hours. Engages in repetitive behavior. Spoon fed.

11/71: Psychiatrist prescribes medication for client to control repetitive behaviors. Client does not speak, appears totally unaware of surroundings.

12/71: Client transferred to acute care wing, where he is fed, toileted, and moved.

1/73: Today I close my file on Isadore Rose. Client deceased.

It took me 10 years to understand what had happened to Isadore Rose. I had never empathized with him, nor with the scores of very old people like him with whom I worked from 1963 to 1973. I judged them by standards that applied to much younger people, people who had not suffered the physical and social losses of very old age, people who had faced their emotions along the way, people who did not have to express unfinished feelings in order to die in peace. Isadore Rose's eyesight and hearing were impaired. He suffered from a weak bladder and damaged brain cells and could no longer control his anger in old age. He could not "listen to reason" and conform to my sense of reality. He was not motivated to calm down and modify his behavior. He needed to yell, to rid himself of his bottled-up rage. He had his own reality. He was using his mind's eye to return to his law office and punish the judge who had ruled against him on his important law case. He wanted to re-affirm himself, to shout to his father, "I am a good person. You were unfair. You castrated me with words. I am worthwhile."

I wanted Isadore Rose and others in their 80s and 90s to conform to my standards, to remain oriented to my middle-age conception of reality. I did not know that the very old face a very different struggle. It took Isadore Rose's death to teach me to listen to old people who need to return to the past in order to resolve it.

I never listened to Isadore Rose. Only after he died did I realize that I should have looked at how he had lived his life, how he had faced his life tasks, how he had expressed his emotions, how he had dealt with his losses, how he had rolled with the punches. Isadore Rose was restoring the past to resolve it, to heal himself. His behavior was not pathological but age appropriate. He needed empathy. His life history revealed the reasons behind his "delusions." He heard his father with his mind's ear; he saw the judge with his mind's eye. He used his vivid memories to relive the past to justify himself in his old age. He had shuffled through life, muttering under his breath, blaming others when life hurt. He had never expressed his rage until old age. At age 14, he was silent; at age 84, he finally expressed his hurt. He wanted to be loved. He begged for approval. But it was too late. An avalanche of physical deterioration exacerbated his feelings of inadequacy. Despite his strokes, Isadore Rose would not have become a living dead person if I had listened to him. He would have communicated with me until he died.

Isadore Rose taught me that very old people who survive to old-old age loaded with a backpack of unexpressed emotions must unload these emotions before they die. They enter the final stage of life, Resolution. In Resolution, very old people try to tie up the emotional loose threads of their lives before death. In very old age, they face tasks they should have faced years earlier.

A THEORY OF LIFE DEVELOPMENT AND THE NEED FOR VALIDATION

The Stages of Life Development

Many developmental psychologists, most importantly Erik Erikson (1963), believe that different life tasks need to be completed at different stages of life. In infancy, we learn to trust that Mother will never leave us out in the cold. Warm, safe, snuggled against her breast, we nurse, one with the world. A piercing noise jars our ears—the telephone. Abruptly, without warning, torn from Mother, we are alone. In infancy, we know only present time, NOW. In no time, we are abandoned. Hungry, cold, we shiver. Red in the face with fury, we wail. We face our first life task. We must learn to trust that Mother will come back. We will survive the cold, the hunger pangs, the fury, the fear. Mother proves again and again that she will return. The infant learns with constant repetition: I am lovable. Mother will never leave me. I can wait. I can survive the cold, the hunger, the anger, the fear. Mother will not reject me.

If the infant never learns to trust, the child carries a tremendous burden. In kindergarten, the child runs, stumbles, falls, and cries, "You tripped me on purpose!" That child does not learn to look inside to find the reason for the fall, but looks outside for someone to blame. That child cannot be responsible for hard times. That child becomes a blamer. Instead of trusting that they can survive hardships, blamers suspect society of doing them in.

In childhood, our task is to learn control. We get a kick out of following rules. "Mom! Look what I did—I put everything in the potty. Look what I produced. I did the right thing at the right time in the right place.... Dad! Watch! I learned to ride my bike no-hands! Uh-oh! My bike hit a bump!" The child who learned to trust in infancy falls, cries, then picks himself up and starts riding all over again. "Hey! Look! I did it!" That child may fall again and again. But that child will never fall apart. In childhood, we put our infant's trust to work for us.

But if our parents teach us over and over that we must be perfect—never soiling, never spilling, never falling, never crying, never hurting, never forgetting—we fail to master the task of control, and add another load to our backpack. We carry with us to old age the need to keep tight control. We fear exposing our feelings. We keep our fingers wrapped tightly around the handlebars. We hold onto our possessions. We become hoarders.

In adolescence, our task is to cut the cord, to *rebel*. At age 15, our beloved Mother can turn into a wicked witch. Father becomes a dreadful dragon, breathing the fire of awful authority. At age 15, we must fight to separate from our parents in order to discover our own values. We fight to come up with our own identity. We fight those closest to us. We fight to find out who we are. How are we unique? We've learned in infancy that our parents love us even when we fight them. We can risk rebellion. But if we do not have and hold unconditional love from our parents, rebellion is risky. If we fight and disobey the rules, Mother and Father might not love us any more. We will be all alone. We capitulate. We are good. We always do what Mommy and Daddy want. Who are we? We are Mother's good little girl. We are the teacher's good student, the husband's good wife, the boss's good worker. We never learn who we are inside, separate from an authority. The outside world gives us identity. Afraid of rejection if we assert ourselves, we never learn to be ourselves. To be worthwhile, we have to become somebody's something. Without family, without work, we are nothing. The backpack gets heavier as we get older. We become martyrs.

In adulthood, our task is to *get close* to another human being. We search for intimacy. We want to whisper, "I love you." We want to touch without fear of rejection. If we are clear about who we are, if our identity comes from deep inside, we can risk being hurt. We can say "I love you," trusting that we will survive if our love is not returned. We can risk a fall. We won't fall apart.

But if we fail to accomplish our earlier life tasks, we will not reach out for intimacy. If we could never trust ourselves to take our hands off the handlebars as children, how can we trust ourselves to survive the bumps of adulthood? Haunted by the terror of abandonment in infancy, the agonizing embarrassment of failure as a child, the fear of rejection as a teenager, we must stay apart from others. We become isolated. We become recluses.

Our fifth life task, in middle age, is to *roll with the punches*. We watch our wrinkles deepen, our hair thin; our creased skin doesn't fit the bones, the bags won't go away. We look in the mirror. Everything looks like it did 5 years ago, but it's all a little lower. Some of us suffer an onslaught—an avalanche of losses. We lose a spouse, a breast, a kidney, a job. We face our losses. We grieve. We look in the mirror and accept the fact that we will not live forever. We expand our repertoire for living. We add new keys to the piano of our lives. We move on. A wife dies; we find a close friend. A job goes; we accept a volunteer job.

But if we have learned that we must be perfect, that we cannot lose control, then we cannot spill our feelings to anyone. Without our spouse, we are nobody. Without our job, we are nothing. To survive, we deny the impact of our losses. We cannot risk learning new keys. We bang the same key. We hang onto outworn roles. A widower rejects a new relationship—nobody is good enough. A music lover refuses to buy a hearing aid—it's too expensive. An executive ridicules a volunteer job—his time is worth money. We are stuck, unprepared for the next life stage. We cling to outworn behaviors.

In old age, we have to justify what we have done in our lives. It's time to look backward, to sort out what we *were*. In old age, we prepare to die, feeling good about what we have accomplished in life. We die with self-respect, despite our failures, mistakes, and unfulfilled dreams. I wish that I had been a great actress, but I wasn't. Instead, I used my acting skills to become a good teacher. I like myself. Despite my unfulfilled dreams, despite my mistakes, despite my losses, I am glad that I was born. I respect myself. I have integrity. I can compromise. I can accept what I am, what I was, and what I have never become. Life is worth living.

But if we cannot accept who we are and trust that we will be loved when our eyes blur, our hair thins, our recent memory fades, then we fall into despair. Without deep self-acceptance to outweigh an onslaught of losses, we become bitter and begin to despair.

Despair, if ignored, rumbles inside, turning into depression. Depression is an internal temper tantrum. Rage, rebellion, shame, guilt, love—emotions that have been stopped up successfully for a lifetime—fester. Bearing our backpack that becomes unbearable, we move toward old-old age.

Each life stage has its own unique task. Ignored, each incomplete task re-emerges later in life. The task challenges us to pay attention. The task gives us a second chance at a later time. The task persists, following us to very old age. If we continue to deny its existence, if we refuse to face it, the task finds the moment to take center stage. The task waits for old-old age, when our controls weaken. The task waits until we forget our lines. Then the task moves in.

The Need for Validation

Out of my experience with Isadore Rose and others like him, I developed a method of communicating with empathy that has helped old-old people regain dignity, reduce anxiety, and prevent withdrawal to vegetation. My method—Validation—has helped thousands of caregivers of people like Isadore communicate and avoid burnout and depression.

From Isadore Rose, I learned the most crucial characteristic of very old age: developmental history and physical changes are inseparable. I had to look at *the whole human being*, not just the condition of the brain, to understand the reason behind the behavior. Behavior at every age is judged by physical, psychological, and social development. We

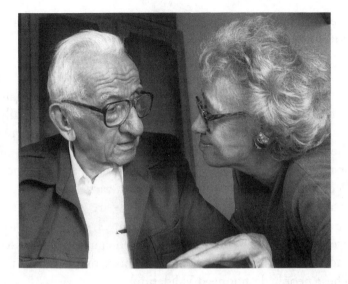

listen to the teenager who vents his rage. We do not judge the teenager by our standards of behavior. We know what it's like to rebel against authority at age 15. It's much harder to empathize with a very old person who has skipped important life tasks and has rebelled at age 90.

Very old age is still new. For the first time in history, we are pressed to understand the old-old, as medicine increases our lifespan. Caregivers face a new breed of very old people who must return to the past to resolve it before death. We must understand the blend of physical, psychological, and social changes that explain the behavior of very old people. A 3-year-old who talks to an imaginary playmate is not hallucinating. He is using his imagination, simulating verbal behaviors, and modeling his parents. At age 3, the behavior is appropriate. At age 33, the same behavior is called an hallucination. At 93, the very old person may be behaving appropriately when he sees someone from the past. In order to empathize with old-old people, we need to understand the complex interweaving of physical deterioration and developmental needs.

Unique tasks are associated with each life stage. People who achieve the life tasks associated with each stage of development learn to master their environments. They gain confidence that they can make mistakes and occasionally lose control without feeling guilty, they learn to express their most intimate feelings without fear of rejection or shame, they learn to trust that they can survive hard times. People who fulfill their life tasks at each stage achieve integrity in late life. In old age, they are able to accept new roles; to grieve over deaths, failures, and unfulfilled dreams; to generate new activity when aging brings losses and familiar social roles change; to move on to new goals. These people do not need Validation.

An increasing number of people reach very old age with some unresolved life tasks. These tasks nag at them, following them to very old age. Incomplete, these tasks re-appear in late life. Buried for a lifetime, these feelings erupt in old age.

People with unresolved life tasks carry heavy emotional burdens that they struggle to resolve in old age. Like Isadore Rose, they use people in present time to substitute for people from the past in order to unload painful emotions. They enter the Resolution Stage of life, the stage in which they struggle to complete unfinished tasks in order to die in peace. Validation is based on the premise that many old-old people enter into this final Resolution Stage of their lives and that certain techniques, described in detail in the next chapter, can be used to communicate with them and help them resolve the past.

In 1963, when I returned to work in The Home for the Aged where I grew up, I found that most of the 170 residents were oriented, integrated human beings who had learned to compromise. They rolled with the punches of old age and still enjoyed living. Only 23 residents had become confused or disoriented. These were the blamers, the martyrs, the moaners, the wanderers, the yellers, the pacers, the pounders whom nobody wanted. I didn't know it then, but each one had accumulated a load of festering feelings. These were the very old people with whom I worked in the Special Service Wing, separated from the oriented residents, who resented their "crazy" behaviors. Staff, too, wanted little to do with these very old people who could not or would not control their feelings and conform. These 23 old-old people would have died of pneumonia or heart disease. But modern medicine kept them alive. They outlived their bodies.

I also worked with the very old oriented residents in The Home. Many of them had survived cancer; heart disease; stroke; and the loss of their recent memory, eyesight, hearing, and mobility. They stayed oriented. In studying their social histories, in talking with their families, in working with them day after day, I found that they carried with them very little excess baggage. They had faced most of life's tasks along the way. They had learned to trust other people, to admit their mistakes. They did not fall apart when problems struck. They were able to express deep feelings. They had survived the losses of middle age and entered The Home prepared for old age. They had compromised. When life wasn't the way they wanted it to be, they accepted things the way they were. They were glad to be alive.

In 1963, the 23 confused residents were diagnosed as having "chronic organic brain syndrome, senile dementia-type, often accompanied with cerebral atherosclerosis." By 1980, the number of disoriented residents had tripled to 69, and they were diagnosed as having "senile dementia of the

Alzheimer's type, with related disorders." As people lived longer, the Special Service Wing for disoriented residents grew. These very old people gradually taught me that they must pack for their final move. They sort out dirty linen stashed in the storehouse of the past. They are busy, irresistibly drawn to wrap up loose ends. This is not a conscious movement to the past. It is a deep human need: to die in peace. Those who achieve integrity in very old age never enter the Resolution Stage. They face their tasks adequately along the way. But, as we live longer, there is a growing number of very old people who fall into the final Resolution Stage of life.

WHO ARE THE OLD-OLD AND WHAT IS DEMENTIA?

Social researcher Bernice Neugarten (1970) distinguishes "young-old" or "younger-elderly" people from "old-old" or "very old" people. According to her distinction, young-old people are between 55 and 74; old-old people are 75 and older. Neugarten believes that the two groups of older adults have different social and psychological needs, and therefore need to be considered separately. I often use the terms "younger-elderly" and "very old" to distinguish the two groups of older adults that Neugarten defined. There are also exceptions as each person ages differently; some 70 year olds act as if they are 90; some 90 year olds act as if they are 70.

Physical Changes Affecting Old-Old People

In my many years of working with older people, I have found that even the most physically fit people begin to experience some physical deterioration after the age of 75. Often, muscle strength decreases; the ability to control the bladder diminishes; arthritis, osteoporosis, and circulatory problems affect mobility; vision, hearing, and sensory acuity become impaired; the blood flow to the brain changes, affecting cognitive function. Arteries that carry oxygen and nutrients to the brain sometimes become clogged, leading to small strokes that often go undetected.

When we reach our 30s, thousands of neurons in the brain begin to die. Unlike other cells in the body, these cells are not replaced. Neuron loss is a gradual process, and by the time a person reaches age 80, the cumulative loss of neurons can be significant enough to affect some cognitive processes, including the retrieval of recently learned facts, dates, and names. Cognition can also be affected by Alzheimer's dementia, a distinct phenomenon that is examined in the next section.

Dementia

The word *dementia* comes from the Latin *dis,* meaning *away from,* and *mens,* meaning *mind.* It was first used in the 18th century by two French researchers, Philippe Pinel and J.E. Esquirol, who used the term to describe mental deterioration and idiocy caused by lesions in the brain.

Identification of Alzheimer's Disease

In 1906, a German neurologist, Alois Alzheimer, examined the brain of a 51-year-old woman on autopsy. Observing "remarkable changes in the neurofibrils… and a peculiar substance in the cerebral cortex," Alzheimer concluded that "we are apparently confronted with a distinctive *disease* process" (Alzheimer, 1907, p. 148). Alzheimer had identified the neurofibrillary tangles and senile plaques that are hallmarks of the disease that bears his name. Neurofibrillary tangles are twisted filaments, or threadlike structures, in the brain. Senile plaques are laminated deposits of a protein, beta amyloid, that is found on the surface membranes of neurons when they degenerate.

The neurofibrillary tangles and senile plaques that cause Alzheimer's disease tend to develop over time. According to neurologist Dennis Selkoe, "most of us who live into our late 70s will develop at least a few senile plaques and neurofibrillary tangles, particularly in the hippocampus and other brain regions important for memory" (Selkoe, 1991, p. 68). Nobel prize winner Carleton Gajdusek reported that 90% of people older than 90 develop plaques in their brains (Gajdusek, 1985). This research has been reconfirmed in recent articles ("Piecing together Alzheimer's" by Peter H. St. George-Hyslop, *Scientific American*, December 2000).

Alzheimer's disease was originally considered a form of presenile dementia. This distinction between senile and presenile dementia was abandoned after 1968, however, after the brains of very old people and younger people were found to be similar upon autopsy. "Senility was renamed Alzheimer's disease, which became a common illness almost overnight" (Miller, 1988, p. 41). Today, the term organic brain syndrome is seldom used, and presenile and senile dementias are not distinguished.

In the most recent revision of the DSM-IV (American Psychological Association's *Diagnostic and Statistical Manual of Mental Disorders*, 1998), Dementia of the Alzheimer's Type (DAT) is listed as the most common cause of dementia and a "diagnosis of exclusion." That means that other causes for the dementia (e.g., vascular dementia, medical conditions such as Pick's disease or Korsakoff's disease, substance induced dementia) must first be ruled out in order to come to this diagnosis.

Jaber E Gubrium, the noted gerontologist, writes:

Diagnostically, Alzheimer's is a disease of exclusion. This means that when a physician is presented with a possible Alzheimer's disease patient, he engages his investigative workup by ruling out other diseases that may mimic Alzheimer's as a dementia. There is a multitude of them. Much of the diagnostic workup, then, concerns the use of investigative techniques that will not pinpoint Alzheimer's disease itself but other conditions that could be causing the patient's dementia.

The accurate assessment of DAT is done through extensive testing (psycho-motor testing and neuroimaging, as well as standard lab work, to mention but a few). Deficits are found in the following areas:

- Memory
- Orientation
- Judgment
- Logical thinking
- Abstract thinking
- Appropriate emotional response
- Attention span
- Performance of activities of daily living

These deficits begin gradually and continue with age. They disrupt functioning in work, as well as on a social level. The decline is much greater than what can be normally expected in the aging process.

The physical evidence of Alzheimer's disease—the plaques and neurofibrillary tangles in the brain—can currently be seen only after a person dies and an autopsy is performed.

The Relationship Between Physical Changes and Dementia in Old-Old People

The relationship between the organic hallmarks of Alzheimer's disease—the neurofibrillary tangles and senile plaques—and the behavioral, psychological, and physical characteristics associated with the disease remains unclear. Neurofibrillary tangles and senile plaques are found in the brains of all people with Alzheimer's disease. They are also found in many people who do not exhibit any signs of dementia or disorientation, however. Therefore, these changes in the anatomical structure of the brain are not the sole cause of changes in behavior in very old people. Many people over 80 survive damage to these brain cells and remain oriented. Although they may have a visual impairment, a hearing impairment, and other physical disabilities, these people retain the ability to communicate verbally, are aware of present time and place, and are able to make appropriate judgments. These people have:

- Faced the challenges and disappointments of their lives
- Tackled the problems of daily living with a sense of hope
- Forgiven themselves and others for their mistakes and failures
- Compromised when they could not fulfill goals
- Continued to respect themselves despite failures, mistakes, and dreams that were not fulfilled
- Survived physical and social losses
- Accepted their physical deterioration, loss of loved ones, and inevitable death

- Maintained a zest for living
- Avoided dwelling on the past, but enjoy reminiscing
- Established new relationships
- Prepared for death by making peace with their loved ones

Oriented old-old people do not need Validation. These people validate themselves.

Since 1956, I have worked with oriented old-old people. Some of these people had physical impairments that damaged their recent memories and affected their control over their emotions. Nevertheless, the old-old people with whom I have worked who expressed their emotions—positive and negative—throughout their lives did not vent their anger inappropriately in old-old age. Despite strokes and other physical disabilities that affected their behavior, they remained whole.

Although the cause of Alzheimer's disease is associated with structural changes in the brain, psychiatrists and neurologists who work with older people have long recognized the effect of emotional influences on memory. "Some of what is seen as senile brain disease may be a massive defense against the reality of old age and death," wrote Kral in 1962. "Stress itself may play a role" (cited in Butler & Lewis, 1977, p. 76).

With loss of friends, family, health, and social status, disoriented old people often lose their motivation to conform to social norms. Their failure to resolve important developmental tasks earlier in life catches up with them in old age. They return to the past to resolve it. These old-old people no longer have the tools to cope with the ever-increasing assaults of aging. As a result, they choose to retreat. Validating them helps them regain their dignity. With Validation, they often return to present reality and respond with focused eye contact, improved speech, steadier gait, and regained social controls.

Recognizing that disoriented old-old people are struggling with a legitimate life task may reduce the chance of misdiagnosis. Whereas confusion in a younger person may represent physical disease, disorientation in a very old person may represent the normal struggle of the old-old person who has lost recent memory and surrenders present-day factual thinking in order to restore the past to heal old wounds before death.

Early-Onset Alzheimer's Disease

Disorientation in younger people with Alzheimer's disease is usually not exacerbated by loss of physical health, by changes in social roles, or by the death or illness of family and friends. I have not been able to find underlying psychological or social reasons behind the disoriented behavior of people with early-onset Alzheimer's disease. Unlike older people with Alzheimer's disease, people in their 40s, 50s, and 60s often fail to respond to the touch or eye contact of the caregiver. They stare blankly into space. Often, in the later stages of the disease, people with early-onset Alzheimer's disease lash out without provocation. Although Validation often momentarily improves the quality of life for these people (as shown in Chapter 7), I have not been successful in using Validation to slow the progression of the disease: the people with early-onset Alzheimer's disease with whom I have worked have progressed to Vegetation despite my efforts.

THE OLD-OLD, DEMENTIA, AND HUMAN NEEDS

Abraham Maslow (1908–1970) was a psychologist who developed a theory about human needs. He said that human beings must first fulfill physiological needs (hunger, thirst, etc.), then safety needs (to feel secure and safe), before striving to fulfill psychological and social needs. He created a hierarchy of these needs, which not only seems to apply to oriented and healthy people, but also to disoriented elderly to some extent (see Table 1). Maslow's pyramid of needs doesn't totally apply to very old, disoriented people, but much of it makes sense and gives us more understanding of them.

Since 1963, I have worked with disoriented old-old nursing home residents who have been diagnosed as having Alzheimer's disease. I have documented their social and

Table 1.   Maslow's hierarchy of needs and how they apply to disoriented elderly

Maslow's	As applied to disoriented elderly
Self-actualization: to realize one's full potential	Resolution of unfinished issues, in order to die in peace
Aesthetic needs: symmetry, order, and beauty	Need to restore a sense of equilibrium when eyesight, hearing, mobility, and memory fail
Cognitive needs: to understand and explore	Need to make sense out of an unbearable reality; to find a place that feels comfortable and where relationships are familiar
Esteem needs: to achieve, gain approval, and recognition	Need for recognition, status, and self-worth; need to be listened to and respected
Need to belong and be loved: to feel affiliated with others	Need to be loved and to belong; need for human contact
Safety needs: to feel secure and safe	Need to feel safe and secure, rather than immobilized and restrained
Physiological needs: hunger, thirst, sex, and so forth	Need for sensory stimulation: tactile, visual, auditory, olfactory, gustatory, as well as sexual expression

Source: Abraham Maslow (1908–1970).

psychological needs in gerontological literature and on film (Feil, 1967, 1972, 1973, 1974, 1978, 1982, 1985, 1989, 1991, 1992a, 1992b, 1992c; Feil & Flynn, 1983; Feil, Shove, & Davenport, 1972). I have learned to understand why they behave the way they do, and I have learned to communicate with them.

I have found that a medical diagnosis of Alzheimer's disease tells only part of the story, that it is impossible to understand a person's behavior without taking into account the person's age, social needs, and psychological needs. After having worked with hundreds of disoriented old-old people, I began to understand their psychological needs. I realized that people who become disoriented in late life have certain psychological and social needs:

- They need to express feelings that have been locked up inside them throughout their lives.

- They need to restore a sense of equilibrium and relieve loneliness when eyesight, hearing, mobility, and recent memory fail.

- They need to restore their former social roles. They often use people in present time to represent significant loved ones from the past.

- They need to resolve unsatisfactory relationships from the past before they die.

- They need to resolve unfinished life tasks in order to die in peace.

To satisfy these needs, they use the mind's eye to see; they recall familiar voices from the past, which sound real to them. To relive the sense of usefulness they experienced when they were working, they move their hands and feet in the same way that they may have done in their jobs. Once they lose the ability to communicate through speech, they blend sounds to express their emotions. Most important, despite disorientation, they keep the universal human need to belong, to find identity, to express themselves.

In more than 30 years of caring about and working with disoriented old-old people, I have found that *when they are validated, when their psychological and social needs are met, they do not regress to Vegetation.* They continue to communicate until they die. Often, dormant speech re-appears; eyes light; gait improves; well-established familiar social roles return; negative behaviors, such as crying, pacing, blaming, and pounding, decrease.

Old-old people who, isolated, try to work through the anguish of Resolution, suffer enormously. They are often a source of frustration and pain to caregivers and family members, who are at a loss as to how to deal with their incomprehensible behaviors. As more and more people in the United States and elsewhere in the world reach old-old age, more and more families and institutions will be confronted with bizarre and upsetting behaviors. The need to find some way of understanding and communicating with disoriented old people is overwhelming.

Caregivers and family members who view very old, disoriented people as simply demented are unable to validate them. However, once caregivers learn to perceive these people as human beings who have deteriorated physically, who are no longer able to cope with the assaults of aging, and who are involved in a final struggle to resolve the unfinished tasks of their lives, caregivers begin to understand. Armed with the simple techniques of Validation, described in Chapter 2, caregivers learn to communicate with disoriented old-old people who are struggling to survive.

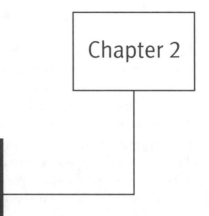

Chapter 2

The Concept and
Techniques of
Validation

WHAT IS VALIDATION?

Validation is a therapy for communicating with old-old people who are diagnosed as having Alzheimer's disease and related dementias. It is a therapy that I developed over a period of many years. As a gerontological social worker, I worked for decades with disoriented nursing home residents. Over the years, I noticed that old-old people with Alzheimer's-type dementia tended to engage in similar kinds of behaviors. Eventually, I identified different clusters of physical and behavioral traits that distinguish different groups of disoriented old-old people. Between 1963 and 1980, I formed a set of beliefs about why old-old people behave the way they do. From this understanding of their behavior,

I developed techniques for communicating with them. Validation developed directly from my experience with old-old residents of nursing homes.

Validation is based on an attitude of respect and empathy for older adults with Alzheimer's-type dementia who are struggling to resolve unfinished business before they die. Validation suggests a way of classifying the behaviors of these disoriented old people and offers simple, practical techniques that help them restore dignity and avoid deteriorating into a vegetative state.

Validation provides disoriented old-old people with an empathetic listener, someone who does not judge them, but accepts their view of reality. As the trust between the old-old person and the validating caregiver grows, anxiety is reduced, the need for restraints lessens, and the sense of self-worth is restored. Physical and social functioning improve and withdrawal to a vegetative state is prevented.

THE PRINCIPLES OF VALIDATION

Validation presupposes the following fundamental, humanistic beliefs and values.

- All people are unique and must be treated as individuals.

- All people are valuable, no matter how disoriented they are.

- There is a reason behind the behavior of disoriented old-old people.

- Behavior in old-old age is not merely a function of anatomic changes in the brain, but reflects a combination of physical, social, and psychological changes that take place over the lifespan.

- Old-old people cannot be forced to change their behaviors. Behaviors can be changed only if the person wants to change them.

- Old-old people must be accepted nonjudgmentally.

- Particular life tasks are associated with each stage of life. Failure to complete a task at the appropriate stage of life may lead to psychological problems.

- Empathy builds trust, reduces anxiety, and restores dignity.

To understand a person's behavior, his or her physical strengths, social needs, and psychological needs must be known. Behavior cannot be judged appropriate or inappropriate unless it is viewed within the context of these needs. For example, a 13-year-old is expected to rebel. Physically, the glands are changing, making it difficult to control behavior. Teenagers swear at their parents, slam doors, and then become contrite. We know that this may be a normal psychological, social, and physiological reaction for a teenager and do not label such behavior as manic depressive. The same behavior in a 45-year-old man, who abused his colleagues and then became depressed, might be diagnosed as manic depressive. Our expectations of a 45-year-old man are different from our expectations of behavior of a 13-year-old. All behavior must be viewed within the context of what is appropriate at each stage of life.

Validation theory and practice is based on the following principles.

1. Painful feelings that are expressed, acknowledged, and validated by a trusted listener will diminish.

2. Painful feelings that are ignored or suppressed will gain strength and can become "toxic."

3. Early, well-established, emotional memories remain on some level into old-old age.

4. When more recent memory fails, older adults try to restore balance to their lives by retrieving earlier memories.

5. When eyesight fails, they use the mind's eye to see. When hearing goes, they listen to sounds from the past.

6. Human beings have many levels of awareness.

7. When present reality becomes painful, some old-old survive by retreating and stimulating memories of the past.

8. Emotions felt in present time can trigger similar emotions felt in the past.

A validating caregiver acknowledges the loss of eyesight, hearing, recent memory, and social controls of very old people. A validating caregiver understands that some very old people with a blurry, present day reality can easily return to the past to retrieve familiar faces. They need to go back to mend torn relationships. The validating caregiver does not judge them as behaving inappropriately. Viewed in the context of physical, social, and psychological factors, their behavior is healing; their retrieval of the past is functional.

Validation is based on the notion that there is a reason behind all behavior. Understanding why disoriented old-old people behave the way they do and accepting the way they behave is the key to validating them. The validating caregiver accepts the physical deterioration of the person; enters that person's world; and becomes a nurturing, trusted authority. The old-old person then feels safe, and begins to communicate, with or without words.

Disoriented old-old people respond to the genuine touching, nurturing, caring, and empathy they feel from the validating caregiver. Increased feelings of self-worth and well-being through Validation often lead to significant changes in behavior. Most importantly, older people in Resolution do not withdraw inward to a vegetative state, but continue to communicate to the maximum of their potential.

THE FOUR STAGES OF RESOLUTION

Very old people who have ignored or denied the need for important life tasks in earlier stages of their life enter a period of their lives in which they feel the need to resolve unfinished business in order to die in peace. They generally progress through four stages of Resolution: 1) Malorientation, 2) Time Confusion, 3) Repetitive Motion, and 4) Vegetation (see Figure 1). With each stage, physical deterioration worsens and there is a progressive withdrawal inward (Table 2). Categorizing very old, disoriented human beings is difficult, however, since people often wander from stage to stage. Each person is unique; there can be no formula for categorizing

Table 2. The four stages of Resolution

	Stage 1 Malorientation	Stage 2 Time Confusion	Stage 3 Repetitive Motion	Stage 4 Vegetation
Basic helping clues (to be used by caregiver)	• Use who, what, where, and when type questions • Use minimal touch • Maintain social distance	• Use "feeling" words (I see . . . I feel) • Use touch and eye contact	• Use touch and eye contact • Pace to person's movements • Mirror emotions and movements	• Use sensory stimulation • Use music
Orientation (of person)	• Keeps time • Holds on to present reality • Realizes and is threatened by own disorientation	• Does not keep track of clock time • Forgets facts, names, and places • Difficulty with nouns	• Shuts out most stimulation from the outside world • Has own sense of time	• Will not recognize family, visitors, old friends, or staff • No sense of time
Body patterns; muscles (of person)	• Tense, tight muscles • Usually continent • Quick, direct movements • Purposeful gait	• Sits upright but relaxed • Aware of incontinence • Slow, smooth movements	• Slumps forward • Unaware of incontinence • Restless, paces; • Repeats early childhood movements/sounds	• Flaccid • Little movement • No effort to control continence
Vocal tone (of person)	• Harsh, accusatory, and often whining	• Low, rarely harsh • Sings readily	• Slow, steady	• No speech

32

Eyes (of person)	• Clear and bright • Focused, good eye contact	• Downcast, eye contact triggers recognition	• Usually closed	• Eyes shut (face closed, lacks expression) • Stares without focusing
Emotions (of person)	• Denies feelings	• Substitutes memories and feelings from past to present situations	• Demonstrates feelings openly	• Difficult to assess
Personal care (by person)	• Can do basic care	• Misplaces personal items often • Creates own rules of behavior	• Cannot care for themselves	• Cannot care for themselves
Communication (of person)	• Positive responses to recognized roles and people • Negative responses to those less oriented	• Responds to nurturing tone and touch • Smiles when greeted • Begins to use unique word combinations	• Uses few commonly used words • Communicates mainly on a nonverbal level • Substitutes movements for speech	• Rare, minimal • Responds occasionally to singing and touching
Memory and intellect rules (of person)	• Can read and write, unless blind • Sticks to rules and conventions	• Can read but no longer writes legibly • Makes up own rules	• Is not motivated to read or write • Early memories and universal symbols are most meaningful	• Difficult to assess
Humor (of person)	• Some humor retained	• Cannot play games with rules • Humor is unique	• Laughs easily, often unprompted	• Difficult to assess

Reproduced by kind permission of Nursing Times where this figure first appeared in an article on February 10, 1988.

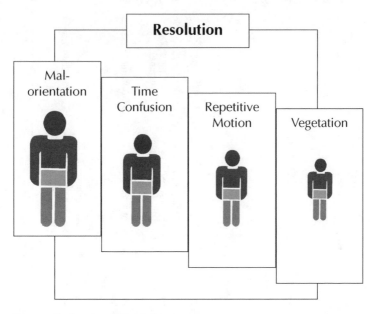

Figure 1. The four stages of Resolution.

human beings. A 90-year-old woman may be oriented at 7:00 A.M. At 8:30 A.M., she may be convinced that a man is under her bed. At 2:30 P.M., she may demand to go home to see her mother. Despite these fluctuations during the day, however, most people stay in one stage of Resolution most of the time. If necessary, the validating caregiver moves from stage to stage with the disoriented old person, using the appropriate Validation techniques.

   Caregivers working with people in the Resolution Stage of life learn to recognize the physical and psychological characteristics of each of these substages (see Figure 2 and Table 2). Chapter 3 presents the first stage of Resolution, Malorientation. Chapter 4 examines the second stage of Resolution, Time Confusion. Chapter 5 looks at the third stage of Resolution, Repetitive Motion. Chapter 6 describes

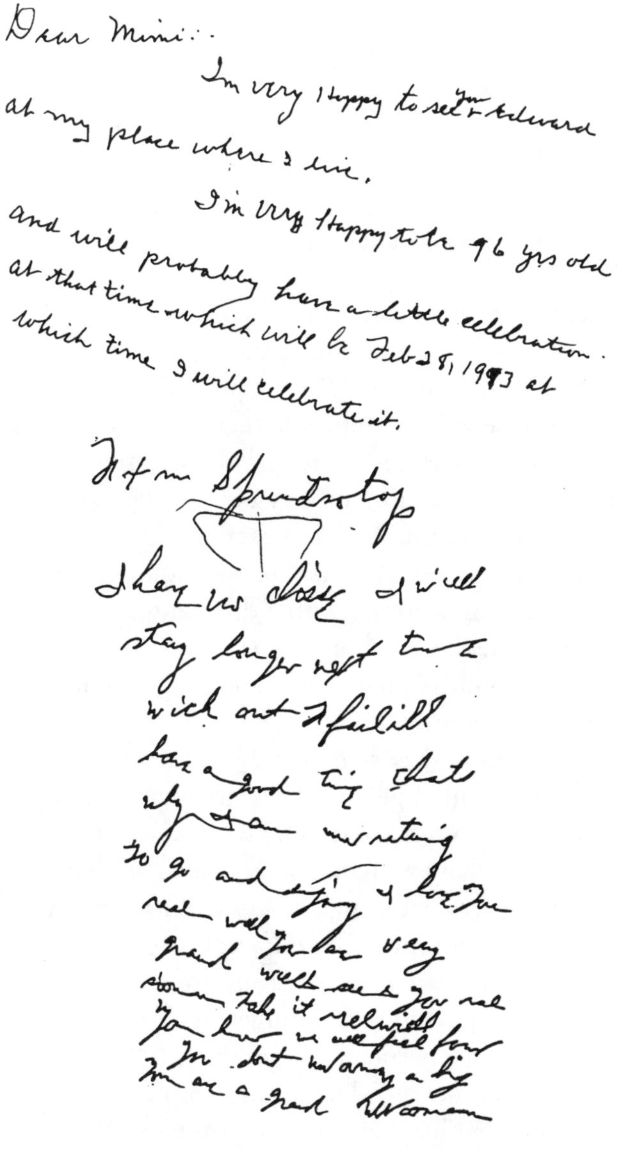

Figure 2. The top writing sample was written by an oriented 96-year-old woman. The writing is fairly clear and legible. The bottom writing sample is typical of a disoriented old-old person moving from Malorientation to Time Confusion. Families and staff can learn to recognize the change in handwriting as one way of assessing the stage of disorientation.

the final stage of Resolution, Vegetation. Old-old people who are not validated can pass through all of these stages. However, as we shall see, people who are validated need not progress to Vegetation and often die at peace with themselves.

THE TECHNIQUES OF VALIDATION

The techniques of Validation are simple. They do not require a college degree, but do require the capacity to accept and empathize with disoriented older people. Validating caregivers must be able to put aside their own judgments and expectations of behavior and learn to be sensitive to the logic behind the disorientation of very old people. Family members, nursing assistants, social workers, physical and occupational therapists, nurses, nursing home administrators, and anyone living or working with a disoriented old-old adult can learn to use these techniques. The techniques require no more than 8 minutes a day of genuine open, nonjudgmental, empathetic listening.

These techniques significantly reduce the anxiety of very old disoriented people. They are enormously helpful to families and to caregivers, who otherwise suffer burnout from working daily with disoriented older adults.

As Chapters 3 through 6 show, different Validation techniques are appropriate for different stages of Resolution. Some techniques, such as Centering, are used with old-old people at all stages; other techniques, such as touch, are appropriate only for particular stages (Feil, 1992b).

The techniques of Validation are simple to learn and can be performed within the course of a typical day. By using these techniques, caregivers can improve the lives not only of the people for whom they care, but for themselves as well.

Technique 1: Centering

To Center, the caregiver focuses on his or her breathing in order to expel as much anger and frustration as possible. By releasing this anger and frustration, caregivers open themselves up to the feelings of the people with whom they are trying to communicate. Since it is crucial to release one's own emotions in order to be able to listen empathetically to another person, all Validation sessions should begin with this technique. Centering takes about 3 minutes and is pleasant and relaxing. To Center yourself:

- Focus on a spot about 2 inches below your waist.
- Inhale deeply through your nose, filling your body with air. Exhale through your mouth.
- Stop all inner dialogue and devote all of your attention to your breathing.
- Repeat this procedure slowly, eight times.

Technique 2: Using Nonthreatening, Factual Words to Build Trust

People in Resolution do not want to understand their feelings. They are not interested in understanding why they behave the way they do. They retreat when confronted with their feelings. To communicate with them effectively, the caregiver must avoid asking questions that force them to face their emotions. Instead, the caregiver should focus on factual questions—who, what, where, when, and how. Caregivers should avoid asking disoriented older people why something happened or why they did what they did.

An 80-year-old woman complains to her daughter that the housekeeper is stealing her jewelry. Rather than argue with her, the daughter concentrates on the factual. "Who is stealing your jewelry, Mother?" she asks. The mother is engaged by the question and responds to it. "That young mealy-mouthed know-it-all. You know—Gladys something or other. I can't pronounce her last name. The one that thinks cleaning a house means moving dust from one room to another."

"*What* does she take?" asks the daughter, continuing to focus on the factual.

"The last things she stole were my black earrings—the ones that Dad gave me."

"Those were your favorite," responds the daughter. "Dad gave you beautiful things. He knew just what looked good on you. *When* did he give them to you?"

"Right after we were married, on our honeymoon," responds the mother. Her anger validated, the mother stops accusing the housekeeper, and begins to reminisce about her husband.

Technique 3: Rephrasing

People in Resolution often find comfort in hearing their own words spoken by someone else. To rephrase, the caregiver repeats the gist of what the person has said, using the same key words. The tone of the voice and the cadence of the speech should also be imitated. In responding to a woman who speaks quickly, the caregiver should also speak quickly.

A 77-year-old man accuses his mechanic of damaging his car. "You broke my gearshift. This is the third time you messed up my car! I'm not paying you one red cent until you fix it! I want my car working the way it used to work."

The mechanic knows that this old man identifies with his car. The gears are wearing out, like the man. The man cannot accept his increasing night-blindness and the loss of his sense of direction. To validate the man, the mechanic rephrases, matching the man's low tone with empathy. "You want your car to be shipshape. You want me to fix it so that it works the way it always did."

"Damn right, I do—no ifs, ands, or buts. Those gears were working fine last week. Now, you fix them the way they were. I'm not buying any new parts for this car. It's a great car."

"You have a fine piece of machinery there, Mr. Simpson. And you say you want to keep it that way. You say those gears were working last week?"

"Well, I was beginning to have some trouble shifting into reverse. When I was driving last night, I almost backed into the wrong driveway."

On a deep level of awareness, the older man knows he is losing his eyesight, and that his sense of direction is failing. He trusts this mechanic, who does not argue or confront him with his losses. Validated, the older man feels stronger.

Technique 4: Using Polarity

The technique of polarity involves asking the person to think about the most extreme example of his or her complaint. By thinking about the worst case, the person being validated expresses his or her feelings more fully, thereby finding some relief. For example, to validate a woman who complains that the food is inedible, the validating caregiver asks, "Is that the *worst* chicken you ever ate?" The caregiver knows that the woman is venting her frustration over her poorly fitting dentures. She knows that the woman needs someone to listen to her anger. By letting her release this anger by complaining about the food, the caregiver helps relieve the woman's anxiety.

Technique 5: Imagining the Opposite

Imagining the opposite often leads to the recollection of a familiar solution to the problem, providing the old-old person trusts the validating caregiver. An 85-year-old woman complains that a man enters her room each night. "That man came back last night." To validate her, the caregiver asks her to think about times when the man does not appear. "Are there nights when he *doesn't come?*"

"Well, come to think of it, when you visited me the other night that man never once showed up. But as soon as you left, and I was alone, there he was—plain as anything."

The caregiver rephrases the woman's words. "You mean, whenever you're alone the man comes. If I were with you all the time, he would never bother you?"

"Well, I was never alone in my whole life. My husband was always with me. It was horrible when he died."

"What did you do after he died?"

"I was so scared that I got all his pictures, and as soon as night came, I took out his favorite waltzes. I stayed up all night looking at his pictures and listening to his music. That's how I made it through the night."

By prompting her to think about a situation in which the man does not appear, the caregiver helps the woman recall how she dealt with a similar situation earlier in her life. Together, the woman and the validating caregiver find the pictures. Together, they reminisce about the woman's husband. The woman restores her familiar way of coping with the fear of being left alone.

Technique 6: Reminiscing

Exploring the past can re-establish familiar coping methods that the disoriented person can tap to survive present-day losses. By the time a person reaches old-old age, it is too late to learn new coping skills. The validating caregiver can help the person retrieve old ways of handling stress, however. By using words such as "always" and "never," the caregiver can trigger earlier memories. For example, by asking, "Did you always have a hard time sleeping, Mrs. Johnson? Even when your husband was alive?" the caregiver may help trigger earlier memories of coping with a problem that the person had since forgotten.

Technique 5, imagining the opposite, and technique 6, reminiscing, are used together. One technique follows the other to help the old-old restore familiar ways of overcoming stress.

Technique 7: Maintaining Genuine, Close Eye Contact

The very old person in Time Confusion and Repetitive Motion feels loved and secure when the nurturing caregiver shows affection through close eye contact. Even older people with impaired vision sense the concentrated focus of the validating caregiver who looks directly into their eyes. Time Confused people who wander, looking for a nurturing parent, often stop wandering when the validating caregiver looks directly into their eyes. The validating caregiver becomes a nurturing parent, and Time Confused people feel safe and loved. Their anxiety is reduced. Often, they will become aware of present-day reality.

Technique 8: Using Ambiguity

Time Confused people often use words that have no meaning to others. They often communicate nonverbally, in ways that are difficult to understand. By using ambiguity, caregivers can often communicate with the Time Confused even when they don't understand what is being said. For example, a Time Confused person may cry, "These catawalks are hurting me!" The caregiver can respond by asking, "Where do *they* hurt?" The pronoun "they" substitutes for the unknown word "catawalks." A Time Confused person may confide, "I wirld with the woomets." The caregiver asks, "Was it fun? Did *they* say anything?" The words "he," "she," "it," "someone," and "something" fill in for the nondictionary words. Time Confused people keep communicating, and withdrawal to Vegetation is prevented.

Technique 9: Using a Clear, Low, Loving Tone of Voice

Under neutral circumstances, harsh tones cause disoriented people to become angry or to withdraw. High, soft tones are difficult for many older adults to hear. It is important to speak in a clear, low, nurturing tone of voice. Often, a nurturing voice triggers memories of loved ones and reduces stress.

A 90-year-old man, Time Confused and in Repetitive Motion, misses his wife. He cannot see, hear, or distinguish present from past time. Looking for his wife in the middle of the night, he finds a sleeping woman and climbs into her bed. The validating nurse understands that the 90-year-old man is returning to the past to fill his need to be with his wife. Although the man is deaf, the nurse nevertheless uses a nurturing, loving tone to ease both the longing of the 90-year-old man and the terror of the female resident.

"Mr. Jones, you miss your wife so much, you thought that Mrs. Drew was your wife. Does she look like her?" she asks in a low, nurturing tone full of respect. As the nurse talks, she gently helps Mr. Jones out of Mrs. Drew's bed.

The old man begins to cry as the nurse takes his arm, helping him back to his own room. "You're a wonderful woman, Molly. You're the tops," he says.

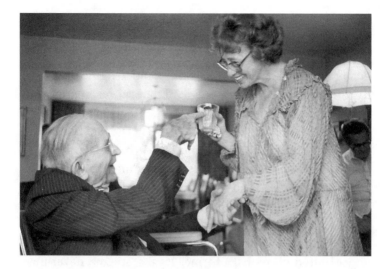

The validating nurse responds in a loving voice, "Molly was a wonderful wife. You love her very much. She is your sweetheart." Together, in a soft voice, they sing, "Let Me Call You Sweetheart, I'm in Love With You." His love for his wife expressed, Mr. Jones falls asleep without medication.

This technique should not be used when the disoriented person is expressing strong feelings and speaking in an emotional tone of voice. Using a warm, loving voice tone with someone who is angry, for example, will only create withdrawal or increased anger. In this case, the Validation worker should match the voice tone—see the following technique.

Technique 10: Observing and Matching the Person's Motions and Emotions (Mirroring)

People in Time Confusion and Repetitive Motion often express their emotions without inhibition. To communicate, it is important to take stock of their physical characteristics and the ways in which they move. The caregivers should observe their eyes, facial muscles, breathing, changes in color, chin, lower lip, hands, stomach, position in the chair, position of the feet, and the general tone of their muscles to match these postures. When the person being validated paces, the caregiver paces. When the person being validated breathes heavily, the caregiver breathes heavily. Done with empathy, mirroring can be effective in helping to create trust. It allows the caregiver to enter the emotional world of the Time Confused person and to build a verbal and nonverbal relationship.

Mirroring the sometimes bizarre motions of disoriented people can be an upsetting experience for caregivers and not all caregivers will want to try this technique. Only caregivers who are truly willing to enter the world of people in Repetitive Motion should attempt this technique.

Mildred Hopkins, a former legal secretary, never married. She worked for the same firm for 45 years. Now, at age 86, in Repetitive Motion, she must keep busy. Work was her only source of dignity. Her brain no longer informs her of her body's position. Seeing her Underwood typewriter with her mind's eye, she moves to the rhythms of her past, swiftly moving her fingers to complete her dictation so that her boss can go to court. The validating caregiver mirrors Mildred's finger movements. Mildred sees the caregiver's fingers matching her own rhythms. She looks up. Their eyes meet. They move together.

The caregiver smiles at Mildred with admiration. "You can type how many words a minute?" she asks.

With pride, Mildred responds, "92."

This was the first word that she had spoken since she entered the nursing home 6 months earlier. In mirroring her movements, the validating caregiver established empathy with Mildred. Secure in the relationship, Mildred begins to look outward. Her speech improves, and she seems more aware of her surroundings.

Technique 11: Linking the Behavior with the Unmet Human Need

Most people need to be loved and nurtured, to be active and engaged, and to express their deep emotions to someone who listens with empathy.

Lovingly, a 93-year-old woman folds her paper napkin. She smoothes out each wrinkle, meticulously wrapping one fold into the other. Nothing is out of place. A waitress who does not understand Validation takes the napkin out of the old woman's hand and shakes it. The old woman begins to yell at the top of her voice: "Help! Help!" Instead of medicating or restraining the woman, the validating caregiver gives the old woman the napkin. Together, they fold it carefully, lovingly, smoothing out each wrinkle.

"Does this make you feel safe and warm?" asks the caregiver.

The old woman smiles. She strokes the napkin moaning, "Ma, Ma, Ma. I love you."

Somehow, the napkin has become a soft, loving mother for this old woman. The caregiver links the folding behavior to the human need for love. When the old-old pound or pace or rub or pat, the validating caregiver links the behavior to one of three human needs—love, usefulness (restoration of movements associated with work), or the need to express raw emotions.

Technique 12: Identifying and Using the Preferred Sense

Most people have a preferred sense. For some people, that sense is vision, for others it is the sense of smell, for yet others it is the sense of touch. Knowing a person's preferred sense is one way of building trust because it enables the caregiver to speak the person's language, to step into the person's world.

To discover which sense a person prefers, the caregiver needs to listen and observe carefully, to try to key in on what the person is saying or trying to say. One technique for determining which sense a person favors is to ask that person to think about and describe an experience from the past. The first sense the person uses often reveals the person's preferred sense. For example, a resident may describe a trip to the mountains she took as a young woman. "It was wonderful," she may say. "We were in the mountains and I could see the tips of the trees." This resident probably prefers her sense of vision and may respond well to visually descriptive words.

Other people may be particularly sensitive to sound or touch and may favor hearing words (e.g., "This sounds bad," "I heard it clearly," "His voice was cruel") or feeling words (e.g., "I feel terrible," "I sense something," "This hits me hard"). To build trust, the caregiver should try to use words that reflect the person's preferred sense.

Technique 13: Touching

Touching is a technique that is usually not appropriate for Maloriented people, but is often effective with people in Time Confusion. The Time Confused have lost their defenses and often have poor vision and hearing. Cut off from visual and auditory stimuli, they need to feel the presence of another human being. They have lost track of clock time and are often unable to recognize people. They no longer distinguish between people they have known all their lives and people they have never met before. The validating caregiver can instantaneously become a loved person, since people in Time Confusion can incorporate strangers into their world.

People in Repetitive Motion are no longer aware of where they are. They are encapsulated in their own space. To communicate with them the caregiver must enter their world and touch them in the same way a loved one touched them. To use touch with a Time Confused person, the caregiver should approach the person from the front, since approaching from the back or the side may startle the person.

I have found that pleasant memories of early childhood are often evoked through touch. With people in Repetitive Motion, the validating caregiver can often establish an immediate intimate relationship by using the following techniques:

- Use the fingertips in a light, circular motion on the upper cheek.

- Use the fingertips in a circular motion with a moderate amount of pressure on the back of the head.

- Use the outside of the hand, placing the little finger on the ear lobe, curving along the chin with both hands, a soft stroking motion downward along the neck.

- Use cupped fingers on the back of the neck with both hands in a small circular motion.

- Use both hands to rub the shoulders and upper back.

- Touch the back of the calf with the fingertips.

Touching another human being is an intimate act, and caregivers—both professionals and families—must always respect that some people, even when their controls are damaged, may not want to be touched. Any sign of resistance to physical contact should indicate to the caregiver that touching is not appropriate. The personal space of all people, whether they are disoriented or not, must always be respected.

Technique 14: Using Music

When words have gone, familiar, early learned melodies return. Stored forever in the brain's circuits, early learning, reinforced through the years, remains. People in Repetitive Motion who no longer retain the ability to speak can often sing a lullaby from beginning to end. When a former sailor, now 95 years old and in Repetitive Motion, paces back and forth, his daughter validates him by singing "Anchors Away, My Boys." The sailor stops, looks at his daughter, smiles, and sings with her. The sailor does not recognize his 60-year-old daughter, nor does he know the name of the song, but he sings each word. His daughter can now communicate with music. She sings with her father because he can no longer talk.

People in Repetitive Motion will often say a few words after singing a familiar song. Music energizes people in Time Confusion and Repetitive Motion.

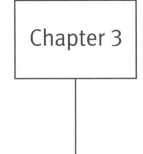

Chapter 3

Using Validation
with People Who
Are Maloriented

The people you will meet in this chapter—and all the people throughout the book—are composites of real people with whom I have worked since 1956. All of the people in this chapter are in the first stage of Resolution—Malorientation. The vignettes show that appropriate use of Validation can help caregivers communicate and avoid stressful encounters.

THE CASE OF FRANCES, THE ACCUSER

Frances Blake was diagnosed with Alzheimer's-type dementia. She was a blamer. She was 82 years old when I met her, and she knew where she was most of the time. She cradled her shiny black patent leather pocketbook under her arm. Frances's pocketbook was stuffed with paper napkins. After cataract surgery and a broken hip, Frances had begun to forget names. It was then that she began hoarding. Hoarding helped Frances regain control. Her purse had become her personality. She filled it up to hold herself together and keep going.

At least once a week Frances would march into my office in the senior housing complex, plunk herself down, and begin to blame. She would always accuse the same person.

"That Elsie Barker did it again!" she would shout angrily. "Last night she stole my pure silk lace panties. Raw silk! Then that hussy marched over to Sam Peltz's room. You know, the good-looking young man across the hall with the mustache! He's only 78." Frances leaned close, cupping her hands to her lips. She whispered to me confidentially, "She stays in his room all night!" She paused for emphasis before adding, "With my panties."

I checked out her story. There was not one shred of truth in her accusations. I showed Frances her raw silk lace panties, with her name sewed in them, hidden under a napkin in her bottom drawer. The more I tried to convince her that no one was stealing her underwear, the angrier she became. Reality orientation made her abusive. Her voice became nasty. "Are you calling me a liar? I know my own pants, and those are not mine! Somebody sneaked those pants into my drawer," she would say when I confronted her. Patiently, I tried to help her by giving her insight into her behavior, to help her understand her feelings, to help her understand why she blamed Elsie.

"Mrs. Blake," I said. "Why do you think Elsie Barker steals your panties?"

"Because that woman is no good! There's a word for her in the dictionary. It's spelled 'w-h-o-r-e.' I don't use that word because I am a lady! I don't fool around with every new man that walks into the building."

"Do you miss having a man around the house?" I asked. "Did you feel robbed when you lost your husband?"

"Just because my husband died, I don't go around stealing other women's underwear," she retorted angrily. "I'm going to let Sam Peltz know what kind of woman that Elsie is."

Frances Blake did not want to understand why she blamed Elsie Barker. She did not want to face her feelings of jealousy. After a lifetime of redirecting feelings she found unacceptable, it was too late for her to change. Blaming had become her way of coping.

Life went sour for Frances after her husband's death; she blamed to survive. Her blaming became so unbearable that her daughter stopped visiting her. "I can't take Mother anymore," she told me. "When Dad died, she blamed the doctor. When she got sick, she blamed the hospital. Now her memory is going. She forgot to turn off the stove and burned the food, so she blamed me. The older she gets, the worse she gets."

Frances Blake never learned to trust herself. She skipped an important life task: to trust that she could survive losses. The deeper the fear, the more she blamed other people. In terror of losing her memory, she blamed her daughter. Out of loneliness after the death of her husband, she blamed Elsie. She ended up alone. At first, her friends tolerated her. They tried to modify her behavior by walking away whenever she began to rant and rave about Elsie. Behavior modification did not work, however; Frances got worse.

Frances Blake wanted to be heard. She needed someone to listen. In her old age, she had reached the Resolution Stage of life. Loaded with feelings she had never expressed, she used Elsie to unload her baggage. She was finally struggling to patch up her life. But we ignored her. And the more we ignored her, the more she whined. Placed on tranquilizing medication prescribed by her psychiatrist, she shrivelled up and was transferred to a nursing home, to become a living dead person in a wheelchair.

Using Validation with Frances Blake

I learned through my failure with Frances Blake. I learned not to contradict, patronize, argue, or try to use logic or give insight. Had I known how to validate Frances, I might have prevented her transfer to a nursing home. When she told me about her stolen panties, I should have rephrased her words by asking "Your best silk pants? When did she steal them, Mrs. Blake?" Feeling my concern, Frances Blake would have begun to trust me.

"Who gave them to you?" I should have asked, to encourage her to reminisce. Mrs. Blake might have expressed her real grief—the loss of her husband and the loneliness of living alone. By validating her grief and anger, I would have helped alleviate some of her stress. With someone to listen to her, her blaming would probably have diminished and she would have been accepted by her friends and neighbors.

THE CASE OF GEORGE, THE LONER

George Smith was another blamer. A fleshy, puffy, 86-year-old man with deep pinkish circles obscuring his small brown eyes, he sat up nights in his overstuffed chair listening for the drip from the ceiling. He would not sleep in his bed. His scratchy voice was weary.

"Can't you patch up that hole? What kind of a man are you? I can't sleep in a bed that's full of water. It smells terrible!"

George's son, James, checked the ceiling. There was no leak. The physician checked George. He found weak bladder muscles that caused George's incontinence. James knew that his father could not accept physical weakness. George blamed a leaking roof to allay his fear of losing control. When his father raised the subject, James tried to divert him.

"Dad, there's no leak in the ceiling," said James. "How'd you like to go out for a cup of coffee and a doughnut? What do you say, Dad, just the two of us?"

"Don't ignore me, James," said George. "You don't believe me. You think I'm making this all up. You don't get dripped on all night. Your roof doesn't leak. You don't know what it's like living here."

George Smith saw through his son's attempts to change the subject, to divert his attention, to ignore his needs. Like all blamers, on a deep level of awareness, George knew the truth. Like a sleeper who, without waking, slaps a mosquito, blamers know unconsciously why they blame. Deep down, George Smith knew that he could no longer control his urine at night. But he could not face this awful truth: the awareness that he was losing physical control over his body was too terrifying.

George Smith had never faced his fears. Throughout his life, he had controlled his feelings of anxiety. He was filled with fears of falling apart. He could not stop the physical deterioration that worsened as he grew older. The worse things got, the more he blamed his son.

At age 88, George was diagnosed by a psychiatrist as "paranoid with delusions of persecution." He was sent to a mental hospital, where he died after 2 years. He had had no previous history of mental illness.

Using Validation with George Smith

I heard about George Smith only after he died. Had I met him earlier, I could have worked with his son to help him validate his father. George's blaming and the son's frustration might have subsided. By using Validation, James could have avoided confronting his father about facts and focused on responding to his emotional needs. The interaction could have been altogether different.

"James, not only did you do a lousy job when you plugged that hole in the ceiling, but you did something to make the pipes spring another leak. I can't tell where the water is coming from. What kind of a plumber are you?"

James would have Centered to free himself of his anger at his father's unfounded accusation and then rephrased his father's words. James would have realized that his father's incontinence was at fault. "You mean there's *another* leak? Where do you think the leak might be coming from, Dad?"

"If I knew where the leak was, I'd fix it myself. I wouldn't ask you."

To help his father express the full extent of his anger and fear at becoming incontinent, James would have used polarity. "How bad is it? How much water is leaking out of the pipe?"

"It's pretty bad, son. And it's getting worse. Do you smell it? The stench is from the sewer, I reckon."

Picking up on his father's use of olfactory words, James might have asked, "Is it a rancid odor? Like rotten wood? Or more like mold?"

"It smells more like mold. The same odor your mother complained about in the hospital. Remember? She used to complain about the old lady in the other bed in the hospital."

James might have realized that his father feared losing control over his functions, the same way James's mother had before she died. George Smith needed to verbalize his fear, indirectly.

James asked, "What did Mother say about the old lady?"

"That she couldn't stand the stench another minute. So, I got her that lilac perfume, the one your Mother liked so much," said George.

"Do you think some lilac after-shave could help now?" asked James.

"Well, we could try it until we can find out where the leak is coming from. I think the pipes are rusted out. We need new plumbing in this house."

James would have understood that his father was afraid that his body was wearing out. George would probably not have stopped blaming the leaking pipes for his increasing incontinence, but with Validation his son would have been able to help his father regain self-respect by validating him whenever he expressed his fear and anger. George Smith would not have died in a mental hospital.

THE CASE OF JENNY, THE GARDENER

Jenny Fish's blaming blossomed when she moved to her new apartment. Jenny was a kind, gentle, 81-year-old lady who worked in her garden every morning. Wearing pink slippers, she gracefully walked down to her rose garden each morning, bothering no one, soothing her bruised roses after a storm. Her problems began when the owners of her apartment building decided to eliminate the garden in order to extend the parking lot. Jenny was forced to say goodbye to her roses and move to a different unit. Six stories up, without even a patio on which to grow potted plants, she began to hear funny noises at night.

"That man next door is banging furniture," she shouted indignantly. "He moves the bed around at night, and he breathes funny. He starts at midnight and goes on for hours so that I can't sleep a wink."

Jenny's apartment faced the outside wall; she had no neighbors. A medical examination found her to be healthy. She had no history of mental illness, no vitamin deficiency, no tumor or kidney infection. Her eyesight, hearing, and recent memory recall were normal for her age. The psychiatrist diagnosed her as "suffering from hallucinations unfounded in present reality, but confined to an imaginary male," and otherwise normal. He recommended reality orientation and behavior modification along with a tranquilizer to reduce her anxiety during sleepless nights.

To reality orient Jenny, her niece, Rita, showed Jenny the wall outside her apartment. Walking up and down the hallway, Rita and Jenny knocked on doors, and found no male tenants living nearby. Hoping that socializing might calm her fears, Rita encouraged her aunt to attend the Garden Club meetings held at a nearby community center. Jenny refused, saying she was too tired to go anywhere because "that man" would not let her sleep. To modify her behavior, Rita excused herself and walked away whenever Jenny began her tirades. Rita's departure made Jenny's accusations worse. The man next door became even more real, taking on a physical dimension. Jenny described him to her one-time friends in vivid detail.

"He's tall," reported Jenny, "with a long nose, huge nostrils, and dirty fingernails. He uses his nails to scrape the wrought iron bed to make that funny sound at night. Don't ask me how he does it, but he breathes that fast panting sound so hard that I hear him right through the wall."

One by one her friends left her. Her niece pleaded with me, "Can't you make her stop? I don't want them to put my aunt in a mental hospital."

That's where she ended up.

Using Validation with Jenny Fish

Had Jenny been validated—by a family member, by an adult day care worker, by a neighbor, by a doctor—I do not believe she would have deteriorated. The scenario could have been entirely different. Jenny's niece, Rita, suspecting serious problems but not knowing how to deal with her aunt, might have taken Jenny to a psychologist trained in Validation. The encounter might have gone like this:

"What does the man look like, Mrs. Fish?" asks the psychologist, focusing on visuals, Jenny's preferred sense.

"He has thick black hair, all over his head and body," she whispers.

The psychologist nods empathetically, acknowledging her fear without words.

"Is he tall?" asks the psychologist, again focusing on the visual.

"He has a long nose with big nostrils, like Jimmy Durante."

"What is he wearing?"

"Doctor, sometimes he isn't wearing anything at all," replies Jenny.

"You mean he is all naked?" asks the psychologist, matching the tempo and pitch of Jenny's voice.

"Not a stitch. Imagine his nerve. Staring at me all night long," continues Jenny.

"What does he do?" asks the psychologist.

"He just looks at me through the crack in the wall. Laughing at me. I think he knows that I hate living in this place," responds Jenny, sadly.

"How long has this been going on?" asks the psychologist.

"Wait a minute. I can't remember the exact day, but I wrote it down in my diary. Here it is. Friday, October 17th."

"Isn't that the day you moved?" asks the psychologist.

"That's right. That's the day they tore up my roses for a parking lot!"

The psychologist, trying to help Mrs. Fish to imagine the opposite, asks, "Mrs. Fish, are you telling me that if you still lived in your old apartment and if you still had your roses to take care of, that man would go away?"

Jenny remains silent for a few minutes and then says, "You know, I never used to see a man staring at me. I was very happy in my own place. I lived there most of my life. And I always had roses, even when I was a little girl at home."

"What kind of roses did you grow?" asks the psychologist. Jenny replies, "They were the most beautiful Peace roses. Very rare in this part of the country. I always bought a special kind of soil for them. Very expensive, but my roses were gorgeous."

The psychologist, suspecting that the fear that Jenny felt when she lost her garden and her familiar home may have triggered her early fears, could have helped her find a creative solution. Jenny needed to grow roses to still her fears. She expressed her love and energy through her flowers.

"Do you think that the man might leave you alone if we found a little spot for you to grow your Peace roses again?"

"It's very likely. Those thorns will frighten him. I think my roses always kept men away. That's why this has never happened before." Jenny feels relieved, and brightens at the thought of gardening again. She begins to trust the psychologist, who helps her find a small garden. Jenny stops seeing her imaginary man. She is able to express her fears to the psychologist, who continues to validate her once each month.

THE CASE OF JUNE, THE BLAMER

June Simpson bloomed as a blamer when she lost her husband. Three years after her husband's death, she tried to shoo away her neighbor's dog and fell and broke her hip. She blamed her neighbor, who had been her friend. "If you had watched that dog, I wouldn't have broken my hip!" she yelled. "It's your fault!"

When her gums decayed, her bridge loosened and she had trouble chewing. She blamed the butcher. "That meat is so tough, only a horse could chew it. Horse meat, that's what you sold me! Now I have to buy a new bridge. I ought to sue you!" The butcher ignored her. Her neighbors avoided her. June, they said, had a loose screw.

June had led a productive, normal, neurotic life. When things went wrong, she pulled herself together by blaming, and then went on with her life. She had been a bookkeeper in a large law office, where she had performed her job with great competence. Before reaching old age, she had never had to face many losses simultaneously. She hadn't developed skills for coping with the multiple problems she now faced in old age, when her losses piled up. She had nothing to do to take her mind off her troubles. She had no one to love. She had lost her husband, had no children, had no job to which to turn. As the pains and losses of aging grew, she found herself unable to survive. Her only way of living through hard times was to blame. She lost her friends and died alone.

Using Validation with June Simpson

I wish I had met June Simpson's neighbors before she died. By teaching them how to validate June, I might have kept her from dying friendless and alone. The brief but unpleasant interaction with the butcher could have been a validating experience for June rather than the bitter encounter it was.

"Horse meat, that's what you're selling me. It tastes terrible. No human being could swallow that meat," screeches June, angrily.

"Does it taste that terrible?" asks the butcher.

"I'll bet you don't eat that meat. You make enough money on us poor people. You can afford the best steak," replies June.

Encouraging June to reminisce, the butcher turns the conversation to June's late husband. "You're used to eating the best," he says. "I remember your husband. He sure knew how to shop. He was a remarkable man."

"He always shopped for me," replies June, her tone already calmer. "Every Saturday. He knew just what to buy."

"What a great man he was," comments the butcher. "He always picked the best cuts. Only filet for him."

"Well, I'll try the same cut. Do you think I should use another kind of tenderizer?" asks June, forgetting her anger.

"It might help," responds the butcher. "How are you seasoning your meat right now, Mrs. Simpson?"

HOW TO READ THE VITAL SIGNS OF THE MALORIENTED

I have introduced you to four very old maloriented people. All of these people suffer in present time in order to express feelings they did not deal with in the past. The validating caregiver does not call them delusional but seeks to ease the pain they feel over these unresolved conflicts. The losses they suffer in present-day reality trigger memories of earlier losses. They blame to cope with so many losses. Their behavior is functional.

What Does it Mean to Be Maloriented?

Maloriented people are usually over 80 years old, have no history of mental illness, speak clearly, and are oriented to time and place, with occasional recent memory lapses. They are oriented, but not happily so. Maloriented people are unhappy because they need to complete an unresolved relationship and use people in present time to express emotions they have not expressed in the past.

- They cannot accept the increasing physical and social losses that inevitably accompany very old age.

- They have never faced important life tasks. These tasks include establishing one's identity; achieving intimacy; learning to establish appropriate emotional and behavioral controls; learning to trust other people; learning to accept losses, especially the losses that come with aging; becoming involved in new activities; achieving integrity; and accepting what is, what was, and what can never be.

- They behave normally in most areas of daily living, but repeat one thing that is often not true in terms of present-day reality.

Physical Characteristics of Maloriented People

People who are Maloriented share certain physical characteristics:

- Their eyes are clear and focused.
- Their muscles are tight.
- Their chins jut out.
- They sit or stand with their arms folded.

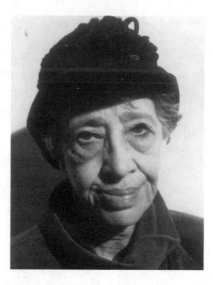

The woman pictured above has the expression of the typical Maloriented blamer. Blamers accuse others to cover their own fears.

- Their body movements are purposeful.
- Their voices are shrill, whiny, or harsh.
- Their speech is clear.
- Their recent memory is largely intact, although occasional lapses occur.
- They retain the ability to read and write.
- Their cognitive abilities, including the ability to tell time, remain intact.
- They experience occasional urinary incontinence.

Psychological Characteristics of Maloriented People

In old-old age, Maloriented people face a final life task. They must express the emotions they have buried for a lifetime. They must finally express fears that they have held for a lifetime. Present-day losses trigger vivid memories of past losses; today's fears stimulate memories of similar fears of long ago. The little boy who was punished and felt ashamed and "bad" for wetting his pants becomes the Maloriented old man who blames his roommate for spilling water all over the floor because he is too ashamed to admit that he can no longer control his bladder.

Maloriented people use people or objects in present time to express feelings that they should have expressed at an earlier life stage. A Maloriented 80-year-old woman who never expressed her bitterness and grief when her husband died at 40 claims that her roommate has stolen her wedding ring. She hides her wedding ring, a symbol of her marriage, so that she can accuse others of robbing her of her husband. In doing so, she finds a way of expressing her anger and grief without coming to terms with her feelings. She does not want to be made aware of the reason behind her behavior. She rejects insight, which frightens her. She does not want to be confronted with her loneliness, which she prefers to deny. These denied emotions cause pain, which she deals with by getting angry at her roommate.

People who are Maloriented share certain psychological characteristics:

- They have no long-term history of mental illness.
- They have generally led relatively productive lives.
- They have failed to complete certain life tasks, and have entered the final Resolution Stage of life.
- They need to express certain emotions that have been bottled up throughout their lives.
- They are unwilling and unable to face unpleasant reality, and thus deny their losses.

- They avoid intimacy and do not like being touched.
- They cling to present time and place.
- They are fearful of losing control of their physical functions.
- They are fearful of losing control of their mental functions.
- They fear change, and adapt poorly to new surroundings.
- They do not want to change familiar behaviors and consequently do not respond to behavior modifications.
- They hold on to familiar coping methods.
- They try to maintain control and deny the loss of control.
- They resist change.
- They are threatened by confrontations.
- They do not want to be analyzed.
- They do not want insights.
- They seek approval from caregivers.
- They feel relief when validated.

Behaviors of Maloriented People

The behaviors of Maloriented people are a result of physical changes as they age and the psychological ways in which they have dealt with crises throughout their lives. Blaming, accusing, whining, and complaining are some of the familiar ways in which Maloriented people cope when things go wrong. They tend to hoard and to clutch items such as pocketbooks, canes, or newspapers. When they reach old age, they cling to these well-established coping methods like a drowning person clings to a life preserver. They are afraid of aging. As more and more things go wrong, their blaming, accusing, whining, and complaining get worse. Maloriented people accuse others of stealing, poisoning, and spying in order to relieve themselves of anger, hurt, or sexual fears. In an attempt to regain control over their lives, they often hoard objects that symbolize their losses. They hoard toilet paper to express their fear of incontinence; they hoard pencils and paper to conceal a fear of losing their ability to write; they hide keys to cover their worry of losing their home or their ability to drive.

Understanding Maloriented People

From 1963 to 1973, I worked with scores of blamers. I spoke with their relatives, their neighbors, their friends. I reviewed their medical and social histories. I began to find clues to their behavior. Similar threads appeared again and again when I pieced together the shabby fabric of their lives.

What clues are revealed in these four vignettes that might help us understand the behavior of these people? All four of these people shared the following characteristics:

- They were diagnosed as being in the early stages of Alzheimer's disease, with paranoid delusions and hallucinations.

- They had no history of mental illness.

- They did not want insight into the reasons behind their behaviors.

- They did not want to change their behavior and were not helped by behavior modification.

- They accused others in order to express emotions they had long suppressed.

- They suffered shame, guilt, and feelings of inadequacy as a result of present-day losses, which triggered similar feelings from the past.

- Without the benefit of Validation, they all deteriorated.

"HELPING" TECHNIQUES THAT MAKE THE MALORIENTED WORSE

People who live or work with Maloriented people and want to help them must recognize what will make Maloriented people worse. I have found that they respond poorly to the following:

- Insight-oriented therapy, such as psychotherapy or counseling

- Behavior modification

- Being confronted with reality when they blame or accuse

- Being helped to get in touch with their feelings

- Being asked to analyze their own behavior

- Being patronized in order to be placated

VALIDATION TECHNIQUES FOR COMMUNICATING WITH THE MALORIENTED

Maloriented people are often well adjusted in most areas of daily living. Their Maloriented behavior is often triggered

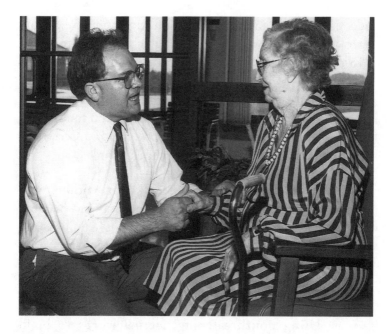

by specific fears induced by aging losses. For example, the woman who sees a man under her bed may behave perfectly rationally until she is overwhelmed by unwelcome sexual thoughts she used to be able to control. A man who is ashamed of his incontinence may behave rationally until he realizes he has soiled himself. He is ashamed and blames others for his faulty plumbing.

Maloriented people respond very well to Validation. A validating caregiver listens with empathy, knowing that Maloriented people are bringing the past to the present to wrap up their lives. When the Maloriented express their feelings of pain and when these feelings are validated, they experience relief and become less anxious. When they are heard, they repeat less often. Listened to with respect by a nurturing caregiver, Maloriented people feel more adequate. After about 6 weeks of consistent Validation, their accusing and whining lessen and often cease altogether. Most importantly, Maloriented people who are validated continue to communicate, and do not deteriorate into Vegetation.

As the cases of Frances, George, Jenny, and June reveal, many of the Validation techniques presented in Chapter 2 can be used effectively with Maloriented people:

- **Centering:** Centering is crucial for working with Maloriented people, whose accusing and blaming behavior is often hurtful to friends, families, and caregivers. Acknowledge your hurt, anger, or frustration over their behavior, and then put these emotions in the closet so that you can tune into the world of the Maloriented person.

- **Using nonthreatening, factual words to build trust:** Use words that get at facts, rather than emotions. Maloriented people are not interested in understanding why they behave the way they do. They are not interested in exploring their emotions. In talking to Maloriented people, use words such as "who," "what," "where," "when," and "how" but never "why"—to get at the facts of the situation. Validate feelings only when the Maloriented person expresses them.

- **Rephrasing:** Repeat in your words what the Maloriented person says, using his or her key words. Pick up the pitch and tempo of the person's voice, the look in the person's eyes, the facial expression. This genuine expression of empathy helps the Maloriented feel understood by a caring authority. Their anger subsides. Rephrasing must be genuine. The validating caregiver corroborates the feelings of the Maloriented and builds trust through rephrasing.

- **Identifying the Maloriented person's preferred sense and emphasizing this sense:** By listening to the Maloriented person, you can identify which sense he or she prefers. If the Maloriented person tends to use a lot of visual words, focus on visual perceptions (e.g., "What does it look like?" "How do you picture it?" "What color is it?" "How tall is he?"). If the Maloriented person reveals that he or she hears noises at night, focus on aural perceptions (e.g., "What does it sound like?" "What kind of noise was it?"). If the Maloriented person complains about feeling pain, use kinesthetic (i.e., feeling) words (e.g., "Is it a sharp pain?" "Is it pounding in your head?").

- **Using polarity:** Maloriented people respond to being asked to describe the extreme form of their experiences (e.g., "How bad does it hurt?" "When is it the worst?").

- **Helping the Maloriented person to imagine the opposite:** Ask the Maloriented person if there are times when the behavior he or she has described does not occur (e.g., "Is there a time when the man does not hide under your bed?" "Is there a time when your roommate doesn't steal your clothes?").

- **Reminiscing:** Explore the past to establish trust and re-establish familiar coping methods that the Maloriented person can use to survive present-day crises. Maloriented people can no longer learn new ways of coping, but they can tap into well-established familiar ways of coping with crises.

To establish a trusting relationship with a Maloriented person, Validation sessions must take place in a private room. The amount of contact time the validating caregiver spends with the Maloriented person depends on the person's verbal capacity, the length of his or her attention span, and the amount of time the caregiver has available. *Three 5- to 10-minute validating sessions a day should be sufficient for people in this stage of Resolution.* To establish a trusting relationship, validating interactions between the caregiver and the Maloriented person should take place at least once a week. It is very important that sessions not be missed, since Maloriented people fear rejection and abandonment. They need to feel wanted.

The results of these sessions should be noticeable. After 5–10 minutes, the caregiver should note the following physical changes to indicate that the Maloriented person's anxiety has diminished:

- The lower lip will be relaxed.
- The voice will be steadier.
- Breathing will become more even.
- The muscles will relax.
- The eyes will be calmer.
- The blaming and accusing stops or lessens.

To end a validating session, the caregiver must remember that most Maloriented people retreat from intimacy. Hugs often make them feel uncomfortable. A handshake or a gentle touch on the forearm is a better way to end.

Chapter 4

Using Validation
with People Who
Are Time Confused

THE CASE OF MARTHA, THE BIRTHER

Here is a portrait of a woman who is still verbal, but who has returned to the past. She is not concerned with present-day reality. She has entered the second stage of Resolution—Time Confusion. The old-old rarely stay in one stage within a 24-hour day. Each person is unique, and there is no formula for human beings. The woman you will meet is in Time Confusion most of the time.

Eighty-six-year-old Martha Johnson grabbed her daughter's wrist.

"Stop it, Mother," Gloria gasped.

Martha's sharp nails dug into her daughter's flesh. Her long, bony fingers tightened as she pleaded, "You've got to get me to a doctor. It's coming out, for God's sake. I have to push. There's no time. Hurry!" Martha clamped her thighs. Her breath came in short, hard spurts.

Gloria pulled herself free of her mother's iron grip. "Mother, you're hyperventilating again. You are not having a baby. You'll make yourself sick. Then you'll really need a doctor."

Larry, Gloria's husband, yelled, "What your mother needs is an undertaker, not a doctor!" He shuffled to the bathroom, his haven from his mother-in-law.

"Take me to Puerto Rico," cried Martha, her fingers clutching the arms of her chair, her teeth clenched. "I can have the abortion there. Get me to the airport!"

Gloria lost control. "You'll be going to a nursing home, not to Puerto Rico. Now quit it!"

Martha shook a bony fist at her daughter, her voice frantic, urgent, hissing. "You ungrateful slut! I have to get to Puerto Rico. I can't wait any longer for the abortion. I'm 4 months pregnant!"

Larry emerged from the bathroom. "Don't you ever talk to your daughter that way. Do you hear me?" He shook her shoulders for emphasis.

Martha's eyes were glued on Larry's zipper. Her face was screwed up with pain, her lower lip caught in her teeth. Her voice was bitter. "You don't care about me. You pretended. Well, I don't care about you. You didn't even pay for the abortion. You son of a bitch!"

"Gloria," cried Larry, "If you don't get that woman out of this house, I'm leaving you!"

Using Validation with Martha Johnson

One month later, Larry and Gloria showed up at my office, where they spilled their frustration. "We can't live with her anymore," said Gloria. "She rarely knows where she is. She keeps reliving some awful memory, something that happened before I was born."

Larry and Gloria told me that Martha had been acting this way for over a year. Gloria had taken her to a psychiatrist, to a neurologist. She had had blood tests, CT scans, all of the latest tests performed on her mother. The doctors had told her that Martha had dementia of the Alzheimer's type. I promised Larry and Gloria that I would meet with Martha.

Martha arrived in my office the next morning. Her hazel eyes darted quickly, searching for something. "Where is it?" she demanded.

I mirrored the look in her eyes. Martha pursed her lips, irritated at my not understanding what she meant. "The operating table," she said. "I can't have the abortion standing up, can I?" She looked at me sharply, sizing me up. "Are *you* going to do the abortion?" she asked. "I don't want a woman doctor!"

"You don't want a woman doctor," I repeated. "Do you think we don't know as much as men?"

Martha tightened her lip, giving me a quick glance. "I know men," she said. "I learned the hard way." Her voice was bitter.

"Did men hurt you?" I asked quietly.

"Why do you think I'm here?" she answered.

I nodded in empathy. "What happened?" I asked, touching her ever so gently on her sleeve. I wanted to know if Martha was more Maloriented than Time Confused. Maloriented old-old people generally resent being touched by strangers. Time Confused people, whose controls are weaker and who incorporate strangers into their world, readily respond to touch. Martha did not flinch from my touch, nor did she avoid the look of empathy in my eyes. If she were Maloriented, she would skirt questions that invaded her privacy. She would not expose her feelings. She would change the subject or tell me to stop asking her so many questions. If she were Maloriented, she would protect herself from intimacy. Instead, she opened up completely, her eyes blurring with tears when they met mine. She held my hand tight and cried.

"He came to fix our radiator. My parents were away on vacation. I have to go to Puerto Rico. You know why. I can never tell my parents. They would be so ashamed," she said. "I'm so ashamed of myself. And I'm so scared."

I nodded, as Martha tightened her hold on my hand. She looked at me as one would look at a close friend. Martha was in Time Confusion, moving back and forth in time. She had lost some cognitive ability. I tried to mirror her feelings of shame by remembering a time in my life when I, too, had been ashamed. I recalled my shame at being the only wallflower at a dance in high school. My tone of voice reflected the feelings I had then. "Were you too ashamed to tell anyone?"

Martha lowered her head and mumbled, "Yes."

"You carried that shame your whole life?" I asked her.

Martha looked up at me, nodding. Her voice cracked. "I didn't tell anyone," she said. "Not my husband, not my children." We looked at each other for a moment in silence. Gently, I stroked Martha's cheeks with the palm of my hand. Martha smiled at me sadly and proceeded to tell me about her abortion.

Martha's shoulders shook with fear, and she tightened her hold on my hands as she spoke. "I can hear them scraping inside," she said. "The pain is so bad. It's twisting around. Help me!"

I stroked her cheeks and held her as she sobbed. "Where does it hurt the worst?" I asked, focusing on the extreme. As she began to scream in pain, I used feeling words to focus on her preferred sense.

"Is the pain sharp or dull?" I asked.

"It's a sharp pain, like a knife cutting me."

After a few minutes she pulled back and looked up at me squarely, her face calm and free of pain. "Do you think I should tell Gloria?" she asked. For a moment, she had entered present time. I rephrased her question to help her find her own solution.

"Do you think Gloria can handle it?" I asked.

Martha bit her upper lip and looked at me for a long time. Finally, she said, "When the time comes, I'll tell her."

I nodded.

After our meeting, Martha's behavior improved. Gloria and Larry noticed the change immediately. Martha recognized her daughter, albeit briefly. "She feels a little better," I explained. "But she'll get worse again. It's going to take time. She wants to come to terms with her past, and she needs you to listen. Her mind can't travel back to Puerto Rico all alone. Can you travel with her?"

Larry's voice was incredulous. "You mean she's going to keep calling Gloria a slut?"

I explained to Larry that Martha had probably felt like a slut herself after getting pregnant 60 years earlier. "She is so ashamed of what happened to her long ago," I said. "She felt like a slut then and projects her feelings onto Gloria now."

Gloria listened carefully, eager to know how she could help her mother give birth to the anger, pain, and guilt she had suppressed for 60 years. I helped Larry and Gloria empathize with Martha. I showed them how to validate her by Centering, by using Martha's kinesthetic sense, by rephrasing Martha's statements, by asking specific factual questions, by using polarity.

I explained Martha's need to be heard before she could stop screaming. I told Larry how to Center when Martha accused him of raping her, to rephrase her words, and to let her rant and rave. Deep down she knew that Larry was not responsible for her problems, and I knew that her screaming would abate with Validation. I taught Larry and Gloria how to travel with Martha by sharing her emotions, by feeling her anger, fear, and misery. Most importantly, I assured them that Martha would feel a sense of relief once she had shared these feelings, and that her pain would subside.

Larry and Gloria validated Martha for 6 weeks, sharing their experiences in a family support group. Within weeks, the Validation techniques I taught them became second nature.

Martha's pains continued, but occurred less and less often. She no longer accused Larry. She recognized her daughter more often. She never completely stopped ranting and raving, but she was no longer abusive to her daughter.

Martha died in her own bed, at age 92. She died peacefully because she had given birth to her feelings 6 years before her death.

HOW TO READ THE VITAL SIGNS OF THE TIME CONFUSED

Time Confused people are usually in their late 70s or older; suffer from increasing deterioration to the brain; have varying degrees of difficulty in walking, hearing, and seeing; and have lost the ability to keep track of chronological time. With Validation, they need not degenerate into Vegetation.

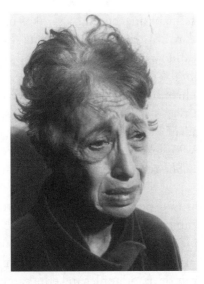

The woman pictured above appears to be in Time Confusion. People in this stage of Resolution blot out the present and use the mind's eye to focus on unresolved past conflicts.

Without Validation, they retreat inward in order to:

- Survive isolation and feelings of abandonment
- Overcome boredom
- Restore feelings of usefulness
- Work through unfinished issues from the past

Because their weakened eyesight has diminished their ability to see, Time Confused people often use the temporal lobes of the brain to restore images from the past. The temporal lobes of the brain also store memories of sounds and smells from long ago, and Time Confused people often hear familiar voices from the past. Since memories that were imprinted earliest are generally retained the longest, older people often recall incidents from the very distant past.

Damage to the brain, caused by strokes or Alzheimer's plaques and neurofibrillary tangles, affects the Time Confused person's ability to think logically and to distinguish the present from the past. Time Confused people no longer keep track of chronological time. They have lost the ability to think in terms of minutes, hours, days, weeks, and months. Instead of keeping track of time, they keep track of memories. A 90-year-old Time Confused woman forgets that she just ate. She remembers only that she must feed her children.

Time Confused people lose the ability to categorize. People with unimpaired brains can identify chairs, tables, and desks as pieces of furniture; they recognize oranges, apples, and pears as types of fruit. Time Confused people can no longer put pears or apples into the category of fruit. Similarly, they fail to distinguish between real objects and those that are merely symbolic. A hand that feels as soft as a baby becomes a baby for a Time Confused woman who needs to be a mother. A daughter becomes a wife to a man who misses his deceased wife.

Physical Characteristics of Time Confused People

Time Confused people share certain physical characteristics:

- Their muscles are loose.
- Their movements are slow and graceful, and they often wander aimlessly.
- Their eyes are clear but unfocused. They often appear to be gazing into space, although signs of cognition appear when they gaze directly at the caregiver.
- Their breathing is slow.
- Their speech is slow.

- Their voices are low.
- They often use their hands to signal their emotions.
- Their shoulders often slump forward, causing them to shuffle.
- They are usually incontinent.

Psychological Characteristics of Time Confused People

Time Confused people share certain psychological characteristics:

- They cannot identify staff and often fail to recognize their families.
- They forget names.
- They mix up people in the present with people from the past.
- They have poor recent memories, but vividly recall the distant past.
- They retreat from reality to escape from boredom and a bleak present-day reality and relive familiar scenes from the past, which they often struggle to resolve.
- They use objects as substitutes for people.
- They are unable to categorize or classify objects.
- They often retain the ability to read, but forget how to write.
- They have short attention spans.
- They remember familiar songs, but often sing off key.

- They are unable to play games with rules, such as Bingo.

- They are unable to control their emotions.

- They freely express their need for love and other emotions.

- They have no motivation to conform to the wishes of their caregivers and often disobey rules.

- They respond to eye contact, touch, and intimacy.

- They retain intuitive wisdom.

- They recognize genuine caring.

- They do not trust caregivers who argue or who pretend to agree with them.

"HELPING" TECHNIQUES THAT MAKE THE TIME CONFUSED WORSE

Time Confused people do not know where they are and usually do not recall how old they are. They are not helped—and may, in fact, be hurt—by constant reminders of their lack of orientation. They are not helped by caregivers who insist that the Time Confused know present-day reality by asking them how old they are, or by asking them what day it is. They are not helped by behavior modification, insight-oriented therapies, or overmedication.

VALIDATION TECHNIQUES FOR COMMUNICATING WITH THE TIME CONFUSED

Validation is crucial for people in Time Confusion. When they are validated, *people in Time Confusion continue to communicate and do not deteriorate into the next stage of Resolution, Repetitive Motion.*

Time Confused old-old people respond to both verbal and nonverbal Validation helping techniques, since they often move from one stage to another throughout the day. They can travel from momentary orientation to Time Confusion then to Repetitive Motion, sometimes within 5 minutes. However, they are in Time Confusion most of the time.

Thirteen basic Validation techniques to communicate with Time Confused people are:

1. **Centering:** Time Confused people can be demanding, irritating, and frustrating. They often vent anger, sexual feelings, and grief. Validating caregivers must Center themselves before they can accept the emotions of the Time Confused. Breathing deeply helps caregivers release their own negative emotions.

2. **Using nonthreatening, factual words to build trust:** Use words such as "who," "what," "where," "when," and "how"—but never "why"—to get at the facts of a situation.

3. **Rephrasing:** Repeat what the Time Confused person says, using his or her key words.

4. **Using polarity:** Time Confused people who have difficulty communicating with words will respond to questions that ask them to relate to the worst or the best. Their attention span often increases when they talk about the extreme.

5. **Using direct, prolonged eye contact:** Time Confused people with little energy respond immediately to empathetic, focused eye contact. Caring is communicated through the eyes. Time Confused people feel

nurtured and safe. They often begin to talk after a moment of genuine eye contact. For Time Confused people in wheelchairs, the caregiver should bend or sit down.

6. **Using ambiguity to respond to a person who fails to make sense:** Time Confused people often create their own words. If a person uses an invented word, use a vague pronoun (e.g., "he," "she," "it," "someone") to respond. For example, a response to a person who says, "These tips don't felangle" might be, "They don't work? Did something go wrong?"

7. **Using a clear, low, warm, loving tone of voice:** Use your diaphragm to project a clear, nurturing voice. Adjust your tone of voice to correspond to the person's emotions. Time Confused people search for a loving parent. When the validator's voice reflects concern and love, the Time Confused will open their eyes, and communication can begin.

8. **Observing and matching the person's emotions:** Observe the person's eyes, lower lip, breathing, hands, and feet. Time Confused people will resist the caregiver who asks them to conform to rules, or to behave in a certain way. When the caregiver observes the facial expressions of the Time Confused and matches their emotions, Time Confused people feel safe and will then move with the caregiver.

9. **Linking the behavior to the need:** Time Confused people express three basic needs: the need to be loved, the need to be useful, and the need to express feelings. A former salesman who is now 90 years old and Time

Confused packs his suitcase every day. The validating caregiver relates this behavior to his need and asks, "Do you want to get on the road, Mr. Jones? What do you sell?"

10. **Identifying the Time Confused person's preferred sense and emphasize that sense:** To validate a person who frequently complains about the food, the caregiver should use words that evoke taste. "What does the food taste like, Mrs. Martin? Is it bitter? Is it too bland? When you were younger, did you like sweets? Did you do much baking?"

11. **Using touch:** Unlike Maloriented people, Time Confused people are not afraid to be touched. They have lost their defenses and respond to a caregiver only if the caregiver is physically close to them. By touching a Time Confused person in the same way that he or she was touched by loved ones as a child, the validating caregiver rekindles memories of a happier time.

12. **Using voice, touch, and eye contact to stimulate a response:** The combination of touch, genuine eye contact, and a nurturing voice tone often sparks dormant speech. Nouns, adjectives, and verbs often will increase (Feil, 1978, 1985; Fritz, 1986). Caregivers have found that touching very old disoriented people often kindles memories from long ago. These early, emotionally tinged memories are permanently stored in their brains and are sometimes stimulated by gentle touching (Feil, 1992b). When touched, the very old person's eyes begin to light; gait and speech improve. People in Time Confusion and Repetitive Motion may begin to talk when the validating caregiver's touch reminds them of their

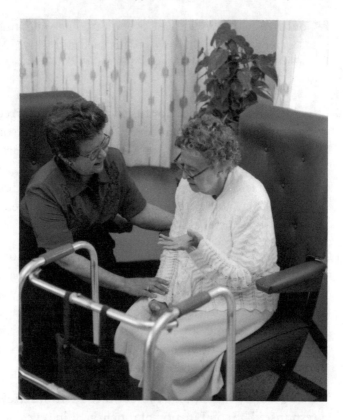

mother's touch, their father's hug, a child's soft hand, or a loved one's caress. When the validating caregiver gently touches the old person's cheek and asks in a soft, nurturing voice, "Is it your mother? Do you miss her?" a disoriented old-old person will often respond with words.

In the 1978 documentary "Looking for Yesterday" (Feil, 1978), a caregiver touches an 86-year-old woman, Mrs. Kessler. For the first time in months, Mrs. Kessler opens her eyes, looks directly at the caregiver, and says, "I love my mother. She is the prettiest in the city." Within 5 minutes, Mrs. Kessler progresses from Repetitive Motion to Time Confusion to awareness of present-day reality, as the caregiver's touch stimulates feelings of safety.

13. **Using music:** Songs learned in early childhood become permanently imprinted on the brain. Time Confused people who no longer recognize people and who are losing the ability to speak often remember songs.

A nonverbal, trusting relationship can be established with a Time Confused person in as little as 1–5 minutes—much faster than with a Maloriented person. These sessions should take place six or eight times a day. Unlike Validation sessions with Maloriented people, which are best conducted in a private room, Time Confused people will relate to validating caregivers anywhere. A housekeeper can validate a Time Confused person in the day room; a nurse can validate a Time Confused person while she is giving medications; family members can validate a Time Confused person when they visit.

With Validation, the Time Confused will need less tranquilizing medication, will become less angry, will cry less, and will maintain more direct eye contact. They will use more dictionary words. Their gait will improve. They will smile or sing, expressing heightened feelings of well-being. To prevent the Time Confused person from feeling abandoned when a Validation session ends, whenever possible, the validating caregiver should leave them with a nurturing old-old person, with another validating caregiver, or in a group where the person can engage in an activity.

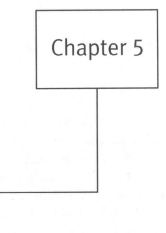

Chapter 5

Using Validation with People Who Are Repetitive Movers

In this chapter you will meet an 88-year-old man who has retreated into the third stage of Resolution—Repetitive Motion. People in Repetitive Motion suffer from degenerative brain damage. They have lost their speech and use movements and rhythms to express their basic human needs. They can be prevented from deteriorating into Vegetation through Validation.

THE CASE OF MARVIN, THE POUNDER

The weary night nurse's laconic smile masked her frustration. Anxious to get home, she muttered to her replacement, "I called Dr. Morgan about Marvin Tubin. He says not to give him more tranquilizers. That's easy for him to say! He doesn't have to listen to that pounding! It'll take all day to get his pounding out of my head. Goodbye!" She slammed the phone. The abrupt thump jived with Marvin Tubin's eternal tapping, ratatat .. ratatatatatat ... rattatat!

The LPN smiled. "The orchestra is warming up." Humming the theme from "Carmen," she harmonized with Marvin's monotonous thumping beat. "Toriodore!" Her strident voice blended with Marvin's pounding.

"Don't spit on the floor. Use the cuspidor. What do you think it's for, eh?" Eighty-eight-year-old Helen Watsall cackled, her shrill voice chiming in. She urged her gerichair closer to the nursing station, pummeling her heels on the floor to gain speed. "C'mon, Silver. Hey, girlie," Helen hissed to the humming LPN, "The old crocker is peeing on the floor. Where's the cuspidor? Eh? Eh? Bubble, bubble, there's the puddle!" Helen, a former English teacher, pointed to the urine seeping innocently under Marvin's chair. She convulsed with giggles.

"Oh, dear," moaned the LPN, following Helen's finger, "they never changed Marvin. He's too heavy to lift alone. I'll wait a couple hours for the orderly." The LPN sighed. She glanced briefly at Marvin, his eyes closed, his face scrunched tight, his fist pounding the flat metallic tray of his gerichair. He was oblivious of his runaway fluids. The acid urine smell filtered through the day room, bothering no one, to be sniffed later only by an occasional visitor. Staff and residents were used to it. Overloaded with charting and medicating, nurses had little time for extra toileting and communicating.

"Whack! Whack!" Marvin Tubin, age 88, slammed his fist hard on the tray. His peppery hair flopped to the rhythm of his smashing fist. Marvin's lips were pursed; occasionally his tongue would sneak between his teeth, helping him to concentrate. Day and night, Marvin Tubin beat his tray.

Without the tray, Marvin beat the palm of his hand, sometimes lacerating his skin and biting his tongue. His fist lay limp, bruised from relentless pounding.

Helen Watsall propelled her chair in front of the LPN, clucking, "Crack. Crack. He broke his back. Better check, honey," the old woman warned, "or there'll be trouble, trouble on the double."

"Oh my God!" The LPN found Marvin's hand black and blue, the skin broken. "Marvin, what did you do? You hurt yourself again. What are we going to do with you? I hate to ask the doctor for more Thorazine." The nurse's voice was soft, caring. She gently touched Marvin on the back of his head, moving her fingertips in a circular motion, bending down for close eye contact. Marvin's eyelids flickered, then slowly pulled wide open, like an old curtain, stiff with disuse. Tears fell slowly, settling in the crevices that ruled his face. His words formed slowly, each letter sounding itself out. "Dad, I got it in straight. Dad, it's only a little crooked. Dad." His voice shook, pleading for approval. Marvin held out his bruised hand to the nurse.

She gasped. She had never heard Marvin speak. His voice was low, rich with timbre. "Marvin," the nurse said softly, bending down even closer to meet his deep brown eyes, clouded with cataracts and tears. Her voice held wonder, admiration, and respect. "You did a fine job. It's in there, straight." The nurse did not know what Marvin was pounding. She used the ambiguous pronoun "it," rephrasing Marvin's words, picking up his pitch. She responded to this old man's longing for approval from his father.

Marvin smiled, his eyes lit with love. "I did a good job, Dad."

For the first time in 9 months, Marvin Tubin responded to another human being. For the first time in 9 months, he formed dictionary words. In the third stage of Resolution—Repetitive Motion, Marvin Tubin no longer knew where he was. His brain no longer informed him of his body's whereabouts. Looking at the nurse, his eyes painted a picture of his father's face. He used his mind's eye to transform the nurse. She had entered his world. Together, they walked through Marvin's past.

This nurse validated Marvin for 3 minutes, four times a day. She used touch; vague pronouns when she could not make out Marvin's meaning; and close, genuine, eye contact. She taught the Validation techniques to the night shift, who were relieved as Marvin's pounding lessened. His dose of Thorazine was lowered. The day nurse sang as Marvin Tubin occasionally pounded a straight nail for his Dad.

HOW TO READ THE VITAL
SIGNS OF THE REPETITIVE MOVER

Old-old people who are not validated when they are in the Time Confusion Stage of disorientation, who receive no stimulation from the outside world, and who continue to deteriorate physically and mentally often retreat to primary, prelinguistic movements and sounds. They withdraw from the world in order to nurture themselves and to meet their basic human need to express their emotions. These people have lost their social controls and are no longer motivated to hide their feelings. In this next-to-last stage of Resolution, they heal themselves by releasing repressed emotions.

People in Repetitive Motion use parts of their bodies, other people, and objects to represent significant people or events from their pasts. A fist becomes a hammer for a former carpenter. A suitcase becomes a briefcase for a former insurance agent. Body movements replace speech as a form of communication. In Repetitive Motion, the old-old lose their self-awareness, a process that begins in Time Confusion. There is a blurring of the self, to the point that old-old people in Repetitive Motion no longer recognize themselves in the mirror. Their feelings spill without reflection. Their emotions pour out in ways that other people find inappropriate. Early learned movements replace speech. Damage to rational thinking frees nonverbal expressions. Motion stimulates emotion. Speech becomes nonintelligible. The lips, tongue, jaw, and teeth move freely to create new words.

There is meaning to the behaviors of people in Repetitive Motion. Although the brain no longer informs these people of their bodies' whereabouts, their memories remain vivid. Memories of early, well-established movements are relived in order to help people in Repetitive Motion survive the bleak reality of the present. These movements are not meaningless, but are ways for people in this stage of Resolution to deal with their losses and to restore some measure of dignity.

People in Repetitive Motion tend to ignore caregivers who disapprove of their acting-out behavior. To validate people in this stage of Resolution, caregivers need to link the behavior to the underlying human need so that they can respond to these needs. As the profiles in Part II show, caregivers who link the behavior to the need are able to validate people in Repetitive Motion, improving their cognition, gait, and social controls, and preventing them from deteriorating into the next stage of Resolution—Vegetation. These caregivers are able to create an atmosphere in which the Repetitive Movers feel safe. The caregivers enter their emotional world.

Physical Characteristics of People in Repetitive Motion

People in Repetitive Motion share certain physical characteristics:

- They are unable to speak in intelligible sentences.
- They repeat sounds they learned in earliest childhood, including clucking, moaning, and chanting.
- They use repetitive movements to express emotions.
- They respond only when stimulated through touch, eye contact, or voice tone.
- Their voices are low and melodic or high pitched and shrill.
- They cry, pound, pace, and rock.
- Their eyes are half-closed or unfocused.
- They move gracefully.
- They are incontinent of urine.
- They lose the ability to read and write.
- They retain the ability to sing.
- They are not aware of the condition of their bodies.

Psychological Characteristics of People in Repetitive Motion

People in Repetitive Motion share certain psychological characteristics:

- They recall their earliest experiences, but have no capacity to retain recent memory.
- They do not remember names or faces.

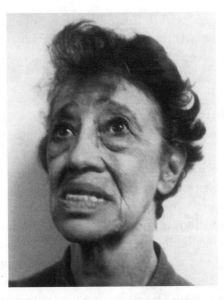

The woman pictured above has the facial expression of a Repetitive Mover. People in Repetitive Motion withdraw inward and use movement to express their feelings after they lose speech.

- They have short attention spans.
- They remember the validating caregiver's touch and voice.
- Their emotions are completely uncontrolled.
- They withdraw from interactions with the outside world.
- They have lost reflective self-awareness.

"HELPING" TECHNIQUES THAT MAKE REPETITIVE MOVERS WORSE

People in Repetitive Motion are not able to stop their movements when asked to do so. They do not understand why they move the way they do and are thus not able to explain their behavior. Asking them to explain their behavior will be unproductive at best, and may be counterproductive.

VALIDATION TECHNIQUES FOR COMMUNICATING WITH REPETITIVE MOVERS

Since people in Repetitive Motion have lost speech, verbal Validation techniques rarely apply. Nonverbal Validation techniques—touch; establishing genuine eye contact; matching emotion; using short, primary words to describe their emotion; linking their behavior to universal human needs (e.g., love, identity, the need to express emotions)—can restore communication. The validating caregiver becomes a trusted, significant person to the person in Repetitive Motion, who incorporates the validator into his or her world. People in Repetitive Motion never learn the validator's name, nor do they recognize their relationship to the validator. Nevertheless, they feel pleasure in this genuine communication.

For the caregiver, frustration and burnout often diminish after just 30 seconds of Validation with an old-old person in Repetitive Motion. The caregiver feels satisfaction as people in Repetitive Motion respond instantly to the validating techniques of mirroring, using music, and matching rhythms. The validating caregiver experiences joy when the use of ambiguity wakes dormant speech in the Repetitive Mover. Mirroring the movements of the Repetitive Mover can spark immediate, direct, genuine eye contact.

Seven basic techniques can prevent people in the Repetitive Motion stage of Resolution from deteriorating into Vegetation:

1. **Centering:** People in Repetitive Motion have lost their ability to think and speak logically. They have lost their sense of self-awareness. The validating caregiver has to enter their emotional world. Validating caregivers must free themselves of their own emotions, so that they can be open to the emotions of the old-old person in Repetitive Motion. An angry, tired, frustrated caregiver cannot accept the feelings of a person in Repetitive Motion. Breathing deeply to Center (described fully on page 37) frees caregivers of their own negative emotions, so that they can Validate people in Repetitive Motion.

2. **Using ambiguity to respond to a person who fails to make sense:** People in Repetitive Motion often create their own words. If a person uses an invented word, use a vague pronoun to respond. For example, a response to a person who says, "These wratches aren't rubbable!" might be "Is there a problem with *them?* Can we fix *it?*" Old-old disoriented people move their tongues, teeth, lips, and jaws, freely blending similar sounds and images to create new word combinations. For example, a Time Confused woman in a Validation group at the Montefiore Home for the Aged combined the words "similar" and "file" to create the word "simofile." Dr. P.K. Saha, the noted linguistic expert who has studied the speech patterns of very old disoriented people, concluded that "nouns, adjectives, and verbs remain in their proper place . . . syntax remains intact. The old-old disoriented form unique word combinations that are not found in the dictionary because of deterioration to logical thinking capacities" (Feil, 1985). This retention of proper grammar and the creation of unique word combinations

by very old disoriented people was first recorded in the documentary film "The Tuesday Group" (Feil, 1972). Since then, Francois Blanchard, Director of Gerontological Medicine at the University of Reims, has videotaped this phenomenon in four hospitals and nursing homes in France.

3. **Linking the behavior to the need:** Like Time Confused people, people in Repetitive Motion express three basic needs: the need to be loved, the need to be useful, and the need to express feelings.

4. **Using touch:** Unlike Maloriented people, people in Repetitive Motion need touch in order to relate. The touching techniques (described on pages 46–47) should be used with people in this stage of Resolution.

5. **Mirroring:** Copy the person's body movements, breathing, hand and feet movements, and facial expressions. Follow the person's lead and dance to his or her rhythms.

6. **Using voice, touch, and eye contact to stimulate a response.**

7. **Using music:** Songs learned in early childhood become permanently imprinted on the brain. People in Repetitive Motion who no longer recognize people and who are losing the ability to speak often remember songs. Speech often returns after singing a familiar song.

Validation sessions with people in Repetitive Motion can take as little as 30 seconds and as long as 5 minutes. These short sessions can be held several times throughout the day to decrease the negative behaviors and to stimulate feelings of well-being. The sessions can end when the pounding, pacing, yelling, crying, or other repetitive behavior lessens and the negative behaviors are channeled into music, movement, or some other activity that meets the need of the Repetitive Mover.

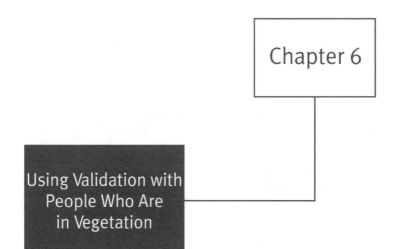

Chapter 6

Using Validation with People Who Are in Vegetation

In this chapter, you will meet a very old human being in the final stage of Resolution—Vegetation. When no one listens during a crisis, when the old-old struggle alone, without Validation, they finally give up. They no longer move. They no longer want. They join the living dead, scattered throughout nursing homes throughout the world.

THE CASE OF NORA, THE NONMOVER

For 6 months she lay inert, curled in a fetal position, her bony, rounded spine poking through the sheets like a pale armadillo. Chin tucked tight in her chest, her threadlike fingers clamped her scrawny shoulders like a vise. Nora Miles took up little space. A few stringy strands of white hair revealed a meager lump of humanity, almost invisible in the hospital bed. Automatically, nurses changed her sheets, toileted her, and turned her to prevent bed sores. Nora never moved, hardly breathed. Dried liquid crusts glued her eyes shut.

Her two daughters had given up 3 months earlier. Until then, they had visited faithfully, once a week. Nora never recognized them. She never spoke. Her lips had disappeared, sucked into her mouth. She had no teeth. Only Millie, a volunteer and childhood friend, tried to spark life from Nora. Millie asked me to help.

"Less than a year ago, Nora's speech was perfect," she told me. Her voice was saddened by memory. "Nora was the happiest of all of us. We were four couples. We grew up together. We were friends since kindergarten—'Nora 'n Horace' . . . they were close. You never said one name without the other. They eloped, both of them only 18 years old. I was their witness, so I went with them to the preacher's house. They loved each other with a passion for 50 years. Nora knew Horace inside out. But Nora never knew about his first heart attack. He made the doctor swear not to tell. Horace died in the bathtub when he was only 68. He never gave Nora notice. I don't think she ever forgave him." Millie's tone was solemn.

"At the funeral, everyone admired Nora. She never shed a tear. Her daughters made all the funeral arrangements. Nora stood straight and tall when they laid the casket. She wouldn't look at him to say goodbye.

"For 10 more years, she strangled her grief. She volunteered with me at the hospital. She kept herself busy, babysitting her grandchildren, sewing for her church. Then she suffered two small strokes. Her recent memory began to go.

The neighbors watched her slip outside in her nightgown in the middle of a wintery night. So her daughters placed her in this nursing home. She did not want to go. She fought like a tiger. She kept screaming that she had to find Horace. They had to medicate her to get her here. It breaks my heart to see her like this."

Millie was a special volunteer. She had given me tremendous insights into Nora's past. Now I had some understanding of why Nora turned inward. She was unprepared for nursing home placement. No one helped her grieve. No one listened so that she could vent her helpless rage. No one validated her feelings. Medication, behavior modification, reality orientation had only made her worse. Eight months earlier, on a wet September evening, Nora slipped past the receptionist, out of the nursing home and scurried down the street. She fell, broke her hip, and landed in surgery.

When she was immobilized, strapped in the hospital bed for 6 weeks, Nora seemed to die inside. She closed down. She no longer called for Horace. She no longer needed restraints. She curled up in Vegetation.

Gently, I touched Nora's neck with my fingertips in a circular motion . . . no response. With feather-like strokes, I moved my fingers from her ear lobes to her shoulder bone. I bent down to meet her closed eyes. Using all my energy, I focused on Nora to spark a flicker of a response. Softly, I sang the love songs that she and Horace must have known so well—"Let Me Call You Sweetheart," "You Are My Sunshine," "I'm Wild About Harry," "Oh! You Beautiful Doll!" Nora's eyes stayed glued. Nothing in her stirred. She barely breathed.

I taught Millie the Validation techniques for a person in Vegetation. With genuine love, Millie validated Nora for 3 minutes, three times every day. One month later, Nora opened her eyes, smiled, and said softly but clearly, "Horace." She died 2 days later.

HOW TO READ THE VITAL
SIGNS OF PEOPLE IN VEGETATION

What Does It Mean to Be in Vegetation?

In Vegetation, the final stage of Resolution, old-old people shut out the outside world, giving up the struggle to resolve their lives. They shut down. Withdrawal is complete.

Vegetation occurs when a person receives too little stimulation, too much medication, and too little Validation. Nora is typical of thousands of living dead people wasting away in nursing homes and hospitals throughout the world: Limp eyelids dropping over closed eyes, hands dangling like drifting oars without a rower, sputum dribbling, shoulders sagging, barely existing. Only the chest moves. No one knows what goes on inside her mind.

People like Nora were not always silent. Their stillness developed gradually, growing day by day as their cries and moans, their repetitive pacing and pounding were ignored too long by staff who were too busy to pay attention to them. In this final stage of Resolution, old-old people obliterate painful present-day reality. They give up the struggle to express their needs through sounds and movements.

Had these people been validated earlier, withdrawal to Vegetation could have been prevented. But ignored, without Validation from a trusted caregiver, with no one to share their inner world, they withdraw. Without stimulation, they begin to vegetate. Once they reach this stage, it is difficult to reach them.

Old-old people in Vegetation differ only in the ways they die. Curled in a fetal position, toileted, turned to prevent bedsores, tube fed, some hang onto life for years. Others die soon after they enter Vegetation.

Physical Characteristics of People in Vegetation

People in Vegetation share certain physical characteristics:

- Their eyes remain closed.
- Their muscles are loose.
- Their bodies are slumped or immobile.
- They often lie in the fetal position.
- Their breathing is soft.
- They are unable to speak.
- They barely move.

Psychological Characteristics of People in Vegetation

People in Vegetation have withdrawn so completely that caregivers cannot identify psychological characteristics. People in Vegetation rarely express emotion and are unable to initiate activity. They rarely respond to Validation.

VALIDATION TECHNIQUES FOR COMMUNICATING WITH PEOPLE IN VEGETATION

Using Validation with people in Vegetation is more difficult—and the results less dramatic—than using Validation with people in earlier stages of Resolution. Knowing the social history of the person is crucial because a person in this stage of disorientation is unable to provide any clues.

The goal of Validation with people in Vegetation is to elicit some facial movement, such as smiling, crying, or singing, and some physical movement of the hands and feet. The following techniques sometimes stimulate nonverbal communication with those in Vegetation:

1. **Centering:** Validating caregivers must focus all of their energy on the person in Vegetation. The Centering technique (see page 37) will relax caregivers, enabling them to focus fully on the old-old person who is in Vegetation.

2. **Using touch:** Caregivers have found that touching very old disoriented people often kindles memories from long ago. These early, emotionally tinged memories are permanently stored in their brains and are sometimes stimulated by gentle touching (Feil, 1992b). When touched, the very old person's eyes begin to light; gait and speech improve. People in Time Confusion and Repetitive Motion may begin to talk when the validating caregiver's touch reminds them of their mother's touch, their father's hug, a child's soft hand, or a loved one's caress. When the validating caregiver gently touches the old person's cheek and asks in a soft, nurturing voice, "Is it your mother? Do you miss her?" a disoriented old-old person will often respond with words.

    If validators know the history of the person in Vegetation, they will know where to touch. If the person in Vegetation had a good relationship with a spouse, touching on the side of the neck with the finger tips can stimulate pleasant memories. People in Vegetation may open their eyes and look, for a moment, at the caregiver.

Touching the check with the fingertips in a circular motion can trigger memories of being touched by a loving mother. Touching the shoulders in a gentle, circular motion can stimulate memories of a sibling or a dear friend. The validating caregiver can touch different parts of the face and shoulders to elicit memories of significant relationships.

3. **Using music:** Music can sometimes stimulate people in Vegetation. Familiar songs learned early in life, songs that have been sung through the years that are associated with loving relationships and strong emotions can sometimes stimulate a response from people in Vegetation.

Contact time with people in Vegetation is seldom more than 3 minutes. A Validation team can structure six very short Validation sessions a day for a person in Vegetation, even if there is no response.

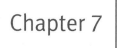

Chapter 7

Using Validation
with People
with Early-Onset
Alzheimer's Disease

In this chapter, you will meet a 62-year-old man whose disorientation was not caused by loss of family, social role, sensory deprivation, or mobility. Damage to brain cells produces the dementia of people who suffer from early-onset Alzheimer's disease. This relatively young man deteriorated despite Validation.

THE CASE OF RICHARD, THE MUMBLER

"Grandpa! It's me, Johnnie! Stop walking away. Don't you remember me? I'm Johnnie!?" The 7-year-old boy's voice pleaded.

"Mayyyyy bee it's the mutterrmublesumble mutterbies," the old man mumbled.

"Grandpa. You don't make sense! Why don't you talk right?"

"Mutterbats mum mummfff." Richard Kraft, age 62, stumbled past his grandson. His eyes vacant, he stared without cognition. He shuffled toward an unknown destination. His shoulders hunched, he bobbed ahead like a ship with sagging sails, drifting with the wind.

"Johnnie! You come right here. Leave Grandpa alone. Do you hear me? NOW! ON THE DOUBLE!" Nancy, his mother, called sharply, her voice shrill. "Johnnie, I want you away from Grandpa." Nancy gritted her teeth, stomping to the living room.

"Mom, look! Grandpa's talking to himself in the mirror again!" cried Johnnie.

Richard Kraft peered at his reflection in the hallway mirror, his eyes blank, his mouth making angry sounds. "Meffle away you mutterstinks!" He shook his fist at the stooped, white-haired handsome reflection. The blotchy, ruddy cheeks were unmarred by wrinkles. "Muddyi maaa musses musss. MUSSSSSTTT!" Richard Kraft roared, bellowed like a lion, and smashed the glass, his fist like a hammer.

"Oh! My God! Why didn't I listen to the doctor and put him in the nursing home?" wailed Nancy. "Johnnie, dial 911. Tell them we need an ambulance right away. Hurry!" Nancy shoved her son toward the telephone and ran to help her father.

Blood dripped from Richard's torn tendon, splattering the rug. Dazed, eyes blank, Richard reeled toward his daughter. Nancy stopped the bleeding. She held her father and her son in her arms and wept, waiting for the rescue squad. "Oh, Dad, I love you so much. Why do you hurt yourself and all of us?"

After placing her father in the Alzheimer's section of the nursing home, Nancy talked to me freely.

"Dad began to act strange when he was only 54," she said. "He'd worked himself up from stockboy to president of the company. And now look at him." Nancy's tone shifted from pride to despair, as she pointed to her father's lifeless form strapped to a gerichair. "That man is not my father. There's no spark. He scares me. His eyes aren't human. He walks like a robot. He used to be curious about everything. He loved living. Mom was a stay-at-home, but Dad took us on trips all over the country. Then, about 10 years ago, his mind started to go. He got worse every day. But Mom would never put him in a nursing home. When the doctor said that Dad had Alzheimer's, Mom couldn't believe that he would lose all of his mental capacity. He kept going downhill. He would put on his coat and start out somewhere, then forget where he was going. He lost his sense of direction. He couldn't tie his shoelaces. Mom would call me often, at 2 or 3 o'clock in the morning, frantic because Dad took the car in the middle of the night. He drove her out of her mind. When Dad wandered or drove the car away, Mom got my uncle to find him. He always found Dad at work. Usually, Dad would be sitting in front of his old building, staring out the window of the car or staring at the wheel. It got to where he never said a word. He wouldn't talk to Mother or me. Johnnie was the only one he related to. They played checkers and read Johnnie's school books. Then Dad began to lose every checkers game. He stopped reading. He didn't recognize my mother. She died last year and he couldn't remember her name." Nancy's voice quivered.

"When Mother died, Dad moved in with us. Dad and Johnnie were buddies until last week, when Dad went crazy.

Dad's deterioration had nothing to do with loneliness or boredom. Something happened to his brain to cause him to lose his sense of reality and his social controls. He was a kind, sensitive, social man. He loved people. I don't want him to die all alone. Can you help me reach him, even if only for a few minutes?"

Nancy watched me mirror her father's body movements. I matched his stride, imitated his gait, and moved to his rhythms. I mirrored his breathing, the downward pull of his lower lip, and the pitch of his voice. Together, he and I shuffled through the long corridors, he mumbling and I singing, "From the halls of Montezuma to the shores of Tripoli."

Richard Kraft had served as a Marine in the Korean War. He tottered a moment, then clapped his heels together, facing me with a sharp salute. "Mumster mafle here." His husky voice was strong, his eyes no longer vacant.

I asked, "Sergeant Kraft?"

"Yes, sir. Present and mimbled, sir." Richard Kraft talked for the first time in weeks.

"Where are you now, Sergeant Kraft?" I wanted to enter his world.

"Can't fuster mums." Richard Kraft's eyes lost luster. He focused somewhere else. He grew blank.

Facing him, I struggled to hold his eyes even though he stared beyond me. "You can't feel them?" I used the ambiguous pronoun to keep communication going.

Richard Kraft turned, ignored my focused energy, shut me out, and shuffled past.

Nancy found three songs that stirred her father. She needed to reach him, to be with him, to love him. Together they would march down the halls, father and daughter, singing, stopping, saying a word or two. But 3 months later, Richard Kraft stopped walking. Within 1 year, he was dead.

HOW TO READ THE VITAL SIGNS
OF PEOPLE WITH EARLY-ONSET ALZHEIMER'S DISEASE

What Does It Mean to Have
Early-Onset Alzheimer's Disease?

Early-onset Alzheimer's disease refers to Alzheimer's disease that begins in a person's 40s, 50s, or 60s. It is fundamentally different from Alzheimer's-type dementia in old-old people because the disorientation is not exacerbated by psychological and social losses. In old-old people the result of disorientation is often a combination of losses and is a coping method that reflects the person's struggle to survive. Unlike the very old, younger people with Alzheimer's disease are not trying to cope by retreating from present-day reality. They see, hear, and move comfortably. They retain a social framework. They do not want to lose contact with present-day reality. They want to keep their social controls and their role in life but cannot because of severe damage to brain structures and brain functions. Their brain damage is usually much more severe than that of a person who becomes disoriented after age 80.

Regrettably, no therapy has been found that is truly effective in helping caregivers communicate with people with early-onset Alzheimer's disease. In older disoriented people, behavior has meaning and represents a struggle to resolve unfinished business. In people with early-onset Alzheimer's disease, I have not been able to discover the meaning behind their apparently random behaviors. Although Validation can offer temporary satisfaction for people with early-onset Alzheimer's disease, it has not been effective in preventing them from deteriorating into Vegetation.

Physical Characteristics of People with Early-Onset Alzheimer's Disease

People with early-onset Alzheimer's disease differ in the emotional lability, the rapidity of their regression, and the length of their lives. They share these physical characteristics:

- Their eyes are vacant and show little sign of cognition.
- Their movements are robotlike.
- They lose speech rapidly.
- They deteriorate progressively to Vegetation.

Psychological and Behavioral Characteristics of People with Early-Onset Alzheimer's Disease

The psychological characteristics of people with early-onset Alzheimer's disease are not known. Behavioral characteristics include the following:

- Their behavior is unpredictable.
- They often hit without provocation.
- They often pace when in a group situation.
- They seldom initiate contact with peers during or after Validation.
- They often do not respond to touch or eye contact.

"HELPING" TECHNIQUES THAT MAKE PEOPLE WITH EARLY-ONSET ALZHEIMER'S DISEASE WORSE

People with early-onset Alzheimer's disease respond poorly to reality orientation, behavior management, excessive stimulation, overmedication, and verbal communication. They are not receptive to logical reasoning.

VALIDATION TECHNIQUES FOR COMMUNICATING WITH PEOPLE WITH EARLY-ONSET ALZHEIMER'S DISEASE

Validation is marginally effective with people with early-onset Alzheimer's disease. Despite Validation, people with early-onset Alzheimer's disease do not improve in terms of speech, social interaction, gait, eye contact, the ability to control emotions or feelings of well-being.

Certain techniques may result in short-term benefits. Adults with early onset Alzheimer's disease often respond to music, mirroring, and occasionally touch.

The Validation technique of using ambiguity to keep communicating with the old-old when they use nondictionary words sometimes helps communication with the person whose disorientation began in his or her 50s or 60s. The speech of a person with early-onset Alzheimer's disease is usually monosyllables, rather than the blend of similar sounds of the old-old disoriented.

1. **Mirroring:** People with early-onset Alzheimer's dementia usually can see, hear, and walk. They will often respond when the caregiver mirrors their movements. Momentary eye contact may occur. A person with early-onset Alzheimer's disease may then imitate the

movements of the caregiver, establishing a nonverbal relationship.

2. **Using touch:** A person with early-onset Alzheimer's disease who is in the later stages of the disease can hit out without warning or provocation. The caregiver should try touching him or her gently on the cheek, back of the neck, shoulders, and upper arm when the person is not aggressive and is in the early stages of the disease.

3. **Using music:** Early learned melodies with emotional overtones remain with people with early-onset Alzheimer's disease. Singing a well-remembered song often sparks a relationship. When the person with early-onset Alzheimer's dementia lashes out, the caregiver can deflect the aggression by singing a marching song.

People with early-onset Alzheimer's dementia require no more than 3 minutes of Validation, eight times a day. Because the younger person usually has more energy, anxiety, and mobility than the disoriented old-old person, the early-onset Alzheimer's person needs more frequent Validation to reduce negative behaviors and to restore feelings of well-being. They need regularly scheduled Validation in a room free of noise or distractions.

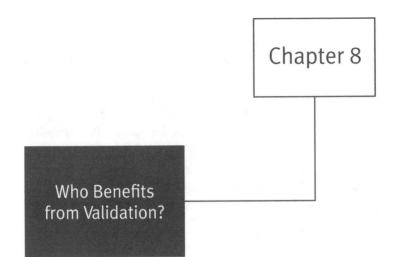

Chapter 8

Who Benefits
from Validation?

Validation helps old-old people who are disoriented as well as the professional caregivers, friends, and families who care for them. Since 1963, tens of thousands of old-old people and their caregivers have benefited from Validation, which has been used in more than 7,000 facilities in the United States of America, Canada, Europe, and Australia.

THE BENEFITS OF VALIDATION
FOR DISORIENTED OLD-OLD PEOPLE

Validation is effective with people who have begun to deteriorate in their late 70s or later, who have lost some recent memory, who have some difficulty walking, who have some sensory impairment, who have lost their position in the mainstream of life, and who are diagnosed as having Alzheimer's-type dementia. These are people who have failed to face important developmental life tasks; who have never learned to trust that they could survive hard times; and who are now unable to cope with the loss of their families, friends, jobs, homes, and health. These are people who have locked up painful feelings inside themselves rather than express them. Now, in their old age, when losses mount, they are overwhelmed. For these people, Validation:

- Restores self-worth
- Reduces the need for chemical and physical restraints
- Minimizes the degree to which they withdraw from the outside world
- Promotes communication and interaction with other people
- Reduces stress and anxiety
- Stimulates dormant potential
- Helps resolve unfinished life tasks
- Facilitates independent living for as long as possible

People who are validated undergo less regression inward; their speech improves; they cry, pace, pound, and wander less; their gait improves; they interact more with other people; their facial expression improves, as they smile more and establish eye contact more often; they communicate more effectively with their families; and they need to be restrained, by physical restraints or psychotropic medications, less often (Alprin, 1980; Dietch, Hewett, & Jones, 1989; Feil, 1982, 1992a; Fritz, 1986; Jones & Miesen, 1992; Kim, 1991; Morton & Bleathman, 1988; Peoples, 1982; Sharp & Johns, 1991).

Validation may not be appropriate for all disoriented older people, and caregivers should be aware of its limitations. Although some caregivers have used Validation effectively with the following groups of disoriented old-old people, Validation was not developed for:

1. Very old people with a history of mental illness

2. People with mental disabilities, such as mental retardation or severe learning disabilities

3. Alcoholics

Documented evidence of the effectiveness of Validation began to accumulate in 1971, when 30 disoriented old-old people at the Montefiore Home for the Aged in Cleveland, Ohio, were studied after participating in a Validation group. These people became more aware of external reality, they communicated more outside of group meetings, and they required less psychotropic medication and fewer restraints following participation in Validation groups (Feil, 1967, 1972).

In another study, the effects of Validation and reality orientation (the basic tenets of which are described in Chapter 9) were compared (Peoples, 1982). This study concluded that "Validation produced significant improvement in behavior . . . whereas Reality Orientation produced no significant difference" (Peoples, 1982, p. 90).

In 1986, a study of the effect of Validation on speech patterns in very old, cognitively impaired, nursing home residents was conducted at the University of Toledo. This study found that "Validation made a significant improvement in the elders' speech patterns" (Fritz, 1986, p. 14).

Researchers at the Irvine Medical Center in Irvine, California, found that "Validation was . . . more effective than application of Reality Orientation . . . . Greater staff awareness of the individual psychological and emotional needs of dementia patients will result in improved therapeutic care" (Dietch, Hewett, & Jones, 1989, p. 975).

Doctors in Australia found that both staff and residents benefited from Validation, with a reduction in withdrawal on the part of residents and more socialization among residents (Sharp & Johns, 1991). Similar results were found in a study conducted at Maudsley Hospital in London (Morton & Bleathman, 1988). In France, Validation was found to promote "an increased resolving of their conflicts and reduced anxiety, less suspicion, and increased trust between patients and nursing staff" (Prentczynski, 1991, p. 7).

In 1993, Robert Gilpatrick, administrator of Child's Nursing Home, in Albany, New York, received funding from the New York State Department of Health and the Bureau of Long Term Care to conduct a 2-year intensive, controlled study of Validation. The purpose of this study is to "evaluate the short term and long term effectiveness of Validation in the management of demented nursing home residents' problem behaviors." A separate team of researchers from the Ringler Institute of Gerontology will evaluate the research.

In the United States, Europe, and Australia, researchers have been able to document the effectiveness of Validation. The experiences of thousands of caregivers, some of which are included in the appendix, confirm this scientific evidence.

THE BENEFITS OF VALIDATION
FOR PROFESSIONAL CAREGIVERS

Professional caregivers of disoriented people—including nursing home and hospital staff and community health care

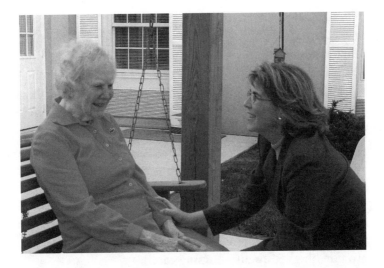

workers who help older adults live independently—often suffer tremendous stress and frustration as a result of their daily contact with people who are disoriented. Validation has much to offer them to relieve the physical and emotional drain caused by working with the disoriented old-old. For caregivers, Validation can:

- Reduce frustration
- Prevent burnout
- Promote joy in communicating
- Increase job satisfaction

A study of the effects of Validation on nursing home staff (Alprin, 1980) found that administrators reported that following in-services in Validation, staff began to view disoriented residents as human beings with intuitive wisdom, not just as mindless bodies. Staff began to understand the meaning behind the disoriented behaviors they witnessed in the facility. As residents responded to Validation, whining diminished and more residents began to speak in adult tones of voice. Fewer residents cried for help. The chain reaction that is often set off when one resident's agitation causes other residents to become agitated was eliminated. The floor was quieter, the facility became a happier place in which to work, and nursing staff began to enjoy their relationships with the residents. Fewer restraints and tranquilizers were used to control resident behaviors.

As a result of these improved conditions, staff turnover decreased 6 months after Validation was introduced. Nursing assistants were more willing to work on weekends and holidays; activity therapists, recreational therapists, occupational therapists, and physical therapists reported increased job satisfaction. Nursing staff experienced less burnout and provided higher quality nursing care.

Nursing home administrators and directors of nursing noted significant changes in staff behavior as a result of Validation. Following training in Validation, nursing assistants in these facilities:

- Called residents by name more often
- Used lower tones of voice in communicating with residents
- Bent down to face residents in wheelchairs in order to establish eye contact with them
- Spontaneously greeted residents more often
- Touched disoriented residents more often
- Toileted and groomed disoriented residents more often
- Communicated frequently with residents' families to share Validation techniques
- Helped residents find lost articles more often

- Listened to disoriented residents
- No longer scolded disoriented residents
- Responded to cries of help from disoriented residents by validating them
- Reported improved relationships with their own parents and grandparents (Alprin, 1980; Feil, Schove, & Davenport, 1972; Prentczynski, 1991; Rubin, 1982)

THE BENEFITS OF VALIDATION FOR FAMILIES

It is not unusual for families to experience even greater frustration than professional caregivers, who are often able to distance themselves emotionally from the people for whom they care. Family members are often angry at their relative for behaving in ways that they cannot understand. Validation has proved enormously successful in helping families communicate more effectively with their relatives.

Families who learn to use Validation often enjoy the following changes:

- They experience less frustration with their disoriented relatives.
- They are able to communicate more effectively with their disoriented relatives.
- They experience relief when their disoriented relatives show improvement in terms of speech and social functioning.
- They visit their disoriented relatives more often.
- They begin to understand their own children better.

- They gain self-awareness as they begin to examine their own responses to aging (Alprin, 1980; Maher, 1992; Ronaldson & McLaren, 1991).

Many of the vignettes that appear in Part II reveal how family members who have struggled with disoriented parents and spouses have learned to use Validation to improve the quality of their interactions with the disoriented people they love.

Chapter 9

How Validation Differs from Other Therapies Used with Old-Old People

The techniques of Validation are based on the beliefs and principles that underlie it. These techniques are tailored to the four different stages of Resolution and differ markedly from those of other therapies used with very old people in the following important ways:

- The validating caregiver never argues with or confronts the old-old person.

- The validating caregiver does not try to give the old-old person insight into his or her behavior.

- The validating caregiver does not try to orient the old-old person to time or place if the person does not wish to be oriented.

- The validating caregiver does not use positive or negative reinforcement to affect the old-old person's behavior.

- The validating caregiver does not use individual or group therapies that require precise rules or orientation to present time.

- The validating caregiver is not an authoritative teacher, but a nurturing facilitator.

Validation is both similar to and different from other therapies used with disoriented old-old people. These therapies—including reminiscence, life review, reality orientation, remotivation, behavior modification, diversion, and psychotherapy—are described next.

REMINISCENCE

The use of reminiscence as a therapy for older adults was first proposed by Mahon, Rhudick, and Butler in 1963. Since that time, it has become an important therapeutic tool for working with older adults.

Like Validation, reminiscence is based on the principle that human development takes places in specific stages, and that managing one's life depends on how one faces the challenges posed by each stage and how one adjusts to the transitions between the various stages. Like Validation, it can be used by individuals or groups of older adults and can be facilitated by trained paraprofessionals. Like Validation, it promotes socialization and mental stimulation and helps older adults wrap up loose ends and restore their sense of self-esteem.

Unlike Validation, reminiscence is rarely useful with old-old people who are in the Time Confusion or Repetitive

Motion stages of Resolution. These people have lost track of present time altogether and live in the past. They are not able consciously to reminisce.

LIFE REVIEW

Life review is a structured form of reminiscence developed by Pincus and Ebersole in 1970. During life review, participants take stock of their lives. As they review their lives, older adults recognize unproductive methods of coping and strive to redirect their lives using more effective coping mechanisms.

In order to undertake a life review, participants must possess verbal skills and retain an attention span that allows them to follow a train of thought. They must be able to put their memories into words and phrases. Some people in the first stage of Resolution may benefit from the reminiscing that is done in life review. However, they may feel threatened when the facilitator of a life review session attempts to give them insight, or asks them to change the way they cope.

People in the later stages of Resolution lack the basic skills to benefit from life review. They will withdraw or become anxious when asked to distinguish between past and present time, or to follow one train of thought.

REALITY ORIENTATION

Reality orientation was developed in 1964 by James Folsom, a psychiatrist working with veterans diagnosed as having schizophrenia and mental retardation. His goal was to rehabilitate his patients with the hope that they might return to the community. His results were promising.

Reality orientation is based on the ideas that: 1) confusion can be prevented, 2) therapy should begin as early as possible, and 3) people feel better when they are oriented to present time and place.

In 24-hour reality orientation, the entire staff of the facility is involved in the patient's or resident's therapy. All staff members who come into contact with the patient or resident use every opportunity to orient him or her with current information. A caregiver greeting a resident might thus say, "Good morning, Mr. Johnson, it's Tuesday, January 5th, and you are in the Fairview Nursing Home."

Where it is not feasible to involve the entire staff, a team is designated to orient the patient or resident. Classes, which can be led by nursing assistants, orderlies, or other paraprofessionals not specially trained to deal with psychiatric disorders, are held daily. Chalkboards, reality information boards, clocks, menus, calendars, and other teaching aids are used in these daily sessions, the aim of which is to orient the participants to present time and place. Participants are gently corrected when their responses do not correspond to present time and place. For example, a 90-year-old woman who remarks that she needs to visit her mother might be told, "You are 90 years old. Your mother is no longer alive."

Both reality orientation and Validation attempt to provide a means for families, friends, and caregivers to communicate with old-old people. The two therapies differ in significant ways, however. Awareness of present time and place is not a goal of Validation, although it is often a side effect as disoriented people become more aware of present-day reality when they feel emotionally safe as a result of their relationship with the validating caregiver. Validation respects the reality of the old-old person, which may or may not be in the present. In contrast, reality orientation insists upon orientation to present-day reality.

Validating caregivers accept old-old people's beliefs and do not disagree with them. Validating caregivers are not teachers, but facilitators. Validation also tries to restore well-being through nonverbal stimuli, including music, movements, and the sharing of feelings.

If reality orientation is nonpatronizing, some people who are Maloriented, who *want* to remain aware of present time, may benefit from it. Such people will not benefit from reality orientation when their belief systems are challenged, however, since Maloriented people often intentionally distort present-day reality in order to restore situations that were unsatisfactorily resolved in the past, or as a coping method to survive losses of aging.

People who are in Time Confusion or Repetitive Motion suffer in reality orientation classes, which make them hostile and anxious.

REMOTIVATION

Remotivation was developed in 1957 by Dorothy Hoskins Smith at the Philadelphia State Hospital. The goals of this therapy were to "remotivate the patient's interest, to get him involved in the world around him" (Jones, 1964, p. 7).

In remotivation, residents or patients meet in a series of meetings held once or twice a week under the leadership of a nursing assistant or other paraprofessional. Noncontroversial topics, such as birthdays, vacations, pets, and hobbies, are discussed. Feelings are not explored, and the emphasis is on factual observations about the present-day world.

Remotivation can be very effective with mildly confused old-old people, like the Maloriented, who may enjoy the interaction with other residents and who are still verbal. The disoriented old-old, whose attention spans are too limited, are often unable to stay on one topic long enough to satisfy the needs of more verbal group members. Their speech is often garbled, they wander from topic to topic, and they are unable to listen to others.

Both remotivation and Validation seek to develop the healthy aspect of a person's personality and to promote the individual's sense of self-respect and self-worth. The two therapies differ in several important ways, however. Whereas remotivation encourages the group to stay on track rather than ramble from one topic to another, Validation encourages residents to talk about whatever they please. Remotivation relies entirely on verbal communication, with the ultimate goal of relating individuals to present-day reality. Validation uses music, movement, and nonverbal media (e.g., balls, rhythm instruments) to stimulate interactions.

Maloriented old-old people may benefit from a remotivation group that sticks to objective topics and avoids dealing with emotions. However, old-old people in Time Confusion or Repetitive Motion will withdraw or become agitated by a remotivation group because of their inability to interact verbally or focus on one objective topic.

BEHAVIOR MODIFICATION

Behavior modification therapy is based on learning principles and the concepts of John Watson. It is based on *behaviorism,* a branch of psychology that studies behavior and observable activities. According to the behaviorists, *learning* can be defined as the relatively permanent change in behavior brought about as a result of experience or practice. Behavior modification is a broad term encompassing many different types of therapies that are used with many different client groups. Assertiveness training, counter-conditioning (to deal with phobias), reinforcement, modeling, and behavior rehearsal are all aspects of this method of changing one's behavior.

Behavior modification, in some form, is used very often with children, not just with the classic toilet-training—reward the child when he or she uses the toilet/potty, ignore or gently scold the child when he or she dirties his or her diaper. It also appears in literature on management of children with attention-deficit/hyperactivity disorder and so-called "troubled teens" with hard-to-manage behaviors. Many self-help books and methods dealing with obesity, smoking, teaching new skills, or eliminating anxieties use behavior-oriented techniques.

The following techniques are used in behavior modification:

- **Continuous reinforcement:** reward after each correct performance.

- **Negative reinforcement:** punishment for incorrect behavior or creating a situation where the client can avoid an aversive situation by behaving properly.

- **Modeling:** allow the client to observe a person with prestige performing the desired behavior.

- **Cueing:** teach a person to remember to act at a specific time, arrange for him or her to receive a cue for the correct performance just before the action is expected rather than after he or she has performed it incorrectly.

- **Some forms of hypnosis:** the subconscious mind is stimulated in such a way as to allow one's body to act on positive suggestions and, therefore, modify behavior.

- **Discrimination:** teach a person to act in a particular way under one set of circumstances but not in another, help him or her to identify the cues that differentiate the circumstances, and reward him or her only when his or her action is appropriate to the cue.

- **Decreasing reinforcement:** strengthen a new behavior, gradually require a longer time period or more correct responses before a correct behavior is rewarded.

- **Variable reinforcement:** an intermittent reward is given after a correct behavior, to maintain an established behavior.

- **Satiation:** stop a particular behavior, allow the client to continue (or insist that she continue) performing the undesired act until she tires of it.

- **Incompatible alternative:** reward is given for an alternative action that is inconsistent with or cannot be performed at the same time as the undesired act.

- **Avoidance:** simultaneously present to the client the situation to be avoided (or some representation of it) and some aversive condition (or its representation).

- **Deconditioning / counter conditioning / fear reduction:** the substitution of a response that is incompatible with anxiety, such as relaxation; the client is first trained to deeply relax, then gradually exposed to the feared situation in greater degrees. This leads to desensitization.

- **Behavior rehearsal:** role playing a difficult situation in a therapeutic situation in order to practice new behaviors.

In modern psycho-geriatric care, behavior modification is used in a variety of ways. Many of the techniques described previously are used by caregivers who want to change the "negative" behavior of disoriented elderly. *Negative behavior* is generally defined as behavior that deviates from society's accepted norms. We naturally apply our own ideas of what is "good" or "bad." Crying, pounding, pacing, expressing anger, and wanting to leave the institution are usually described as "negative." For instance, caregivers reward the resident when she does not cry, with attention and a positive word. Often, crying is ignored in the hope that "if no one gives her attention, she'll stop." Negative reinforcement, in the form of physical restraints or the use of sedatives is often used, although it is rarely thought of as punishment, it is certainly a deterrent. Chiding, scolding, and talking to elderly in a parental manner are used to modify behavior.

Behavior modification requires that the client have cognitive abilities to understand and to remember. As I have described previously, very old disoriented people have lost a great deal of their cognitive ability. Short-term memory is limited. In addition, disoriented old-old people are not motivated to change their behavior in the same way as younger people. The time for change is past. Because of this, behavior modification techniques do not work with the population that is most appropriate for Validation. Sometimes the opposite reaction is stimulated; instead of reducing crying, pounding, pacing, or expressing anger, behavior modification can cause an increase in these behaviors. Sadly, most often the insistence to change behavior causes many individuals to withdraw further into their own personal world and to stop communicating with an environment that offers no understanding or empathy.

In order for any form of reinforcement to be useful, the client must care about the rewards that are offered. An extra dessert, an excursion, or other such offering holds little value to the disoriented old man who wants to be home with his wife or working at his old job. The things that disoriented individuals actively want are respect, a feeling of being worthwhile, to be useful, to be loved, to be included, and to express feelings to an empathetic person who will listen. These are basic human needs that are not compatible with a reward system.

DIVERSION AND REDIRECTION

Diversion and redirection are two frequently used techniques that stem from behavior modification. Diversion is often used to modify negative behaviors. A caregiver trying to divert an old-old person who is behaving inappropriately should provide pleasant distractions once the behavior begins. For example, a resident who is wandering may be distracted by the offer of a cup of tea. Once a person has been diverted or distracted from what he or she is doing, he or she can be redirected to another activity that is more acceptable to the caretaker. In the previous case, after sitting down for a cup of tea, the caregiver may present a newspaper for the resident to read. Such diversion and redirection is temporary, however, because the distraction does not respond to the need that caused the behavior in the first place.

Reading the newspaper does not help the resident express his or her feelings. If no one responds to the resident's loneliness, the resident will continue to wander. A validating caregiver tries to establish a trusting relationship with the old-old person, who, once validated, no longer feels the need to engage in wandering behavior, or feels the need to do so less often.

PATRONIZING WITH THE THERAPEUTIC LIE

The *therapeutic lie* is pretending to believe what a disoriented very old person says is true, even though one knows it is actually false. One lies in order to placate the client. The therapeutic lie arose from a distortion of Validation techniques. Instead of exploring the depth of the old person's personal reality, the therapeutic lie maintains a superficial politeness. It does not take into account the Validation principle—that there are many levels of consciousness. This is the reason why Validation practitioners always tell the truth and are honest. We know that very old people, no matter how disoriented, know what is the truth, who is honest, and who is lying. If we want to develop a trusting relationship with our client, we must be honest and not lie. If we lie, the old person may quiet down but will not trust us. An example from practice follows.

Mrs. Simon, an 87-year-old woman in a nursing home, says in a very worried tone, "Is my apartment all right? I've still got my apartment on Bond Street, don't I?"

The nursing aide responds, "Of course you do. It's still there like always." Mrs. Simon quiets down.

Every day, sometimes several times a day, she brings up the question of her apartment. The actual fact is that her apartment is gone. The nursing aide lied. Mrs. Simon knew on some level that her apartment was gone, and so her worry was not alleviated. Her actual need to be an independent person (possibly the deep fear behind her worry about the apartment) was not met and so the worry came back again and again.

Once we began validating her, and the nursing aide learned not to lie but to explore the meaning behind the behavior, the scene changed.

Mrs. Simon: "Is my apartment all right? It's still there isn't it?"

Nursing aide: "Where was your apartment, Mrs. Simon?"

Mrs. Simon: "On Bond Street. You know, right next to the bank."

Nursing aide: "Next to the bank. Was it a large apartment?"

Mrs. Simon: "Oh, yes, lots of room for entertaining."

Nursing aide: "What do you miss the most?"

Mrs. Simon: "Ah, the friends."

And so the nursing aide explores Mrs. Simon's need for company and her feelings of loneliness instead of trying to placate her with lies.

YOU CAN'T FOOL MILLIE

Here is the story of an 86-year-old nursing home resident who was verbal but Time Confused in Phase Two of Resolution. She needed Validation, not reassurance, therapeutic lying, or patronizing.

Millie Conrad raged incessantly. She swore. "Bitch! Let me out of this hell-hole or I'll piss on you." Millie's green-gray eyes blazed, gleaming with malevolent mischief. She stuck one arthritic finger under Katie's nose. The activity worker bit the inside of her cheek, adding to yesterday's blisters. Millie was relentless. She would not calm down. Each day Katie used her techniques automatically. First, gently confront Millie with reality: "It's not nice to swear, sweetie. You know that. You won't have any friends if you go on swearing like that." Second technique: Redirection. "Look at the clock. Goodness, it's music time! You don't want to miss music, do you? Let's go. Mike is waiting for you. We can't disappoint Mike, can we?" Katie's voice rose, encouraging the old woman. Katie winked at Millie. Sexual innuendo flickered. "You like Mike. He makes you feel good."

Millie stared into space. Her eyes round, now gleaming. Her voice, dreamy: "Harold is waiting? He wants me?"

Relieved that the old woman's rage had vanished, Katie ignored the longing in Millie's voice. Katie nodded furiously, using the therapeutic lie.

"Oh, he really wants you. He misses you when you're not there. C'mon Millie, I'll take you to the Activity Room."

"Okey-dokey!" Millie's high-pitched voice shattered the air. She shoved her hammertoes into faded pink slippers. Katie took Millie's arthritic hand. "Ouch!" Millie yelled and slapped the activity worker's arm. "Bitch!" Millie whistled through false teeth. "That's my bad hand. I told you not to grab. Can't you people remember anything?" Millie muttered in disgust as the two approached the Activity Room.

Katie winked surreptitiously at Mike, the Music Director, and pointed to Millie. Twenty-four-year-old Mike bubbled, fingering his guitar lovingly, waving to Millie:

"Sweetheart, I'm so glad to see you." Mike feigned delight. "You just sit here right next to Sarah."

Millie scowled at 92-year-old Sarah, trapped in a gigantic wheelchair, tubes taped to her nose. Mike's voice hummed: "Now, ladies, take a deep breath before we start."

"That old cow can't even breathe." Millie's voice pierced the quiet as she pointed to Sarah. "Get rid of her. She stinks to high heaven."

"We are all God's children, Millie. We must learn to love each other." Mike's quiet, patronizing voice quieted Millie. She ambled away from Sarah close to Mike, stroking his cheek, peering into his blue eyes, crooning: "I love you sweetie pie. When are we going to get married, lover boy?" Embarrassed, Mike removed Millie's hand, led her back to her chair close to Sarah, ignoring her question.

"All right, ladies, let's start singing 'She'll be Coming Round the Mountain.'" Mike strummed his guitar, his robust voice filled the room. A few weak croaks accompanied him. Six of the 10 women slept. Millie got up and walked away, silent.

That night, Millie's voice pierced the halls of the nursing home. "You son of a bitch! You liar! LIAR! LIAR! LIAR!"

The night nurse tried to shush her. "Millie! You're waking everyone up. Nobody lied to you. Here, sweetie, have a nice, hot cup of tea. You'll feel better. It's rose tea."

"You can take your tea and shove it. Rose tea, hah!" Millie splattered the hot tea on the floor with one furious sweep. "I know when I'm lied to—I'm not stupid. That bastard said he'd marry me. He tricked me."

"Millie, nobody tricked you. Here, take this pill. It'll calm you down."

Millie needed stronger and stronger tranquilizers to calm her down. In 3 months she stopped talking. In 8 months she stopped walking. She lived for 3 more years, a living dead person.

The validating worker may never know that Millie's only love, Harold, abandoned her when she was 16. But, the Validation worker knows that there is a good reason behind Millie's behavior. The old woman was a good girl her whole life. She never married and always cared for her parents. She reached old age friendless. Always controlled, Millie never complained.

At 86, with increasing memory loss, Millie was losing her social controls. Her brain no longer informed her of her whereabouts. She had lost clock time. Minutes, hours, and days lost their meaning. Logical thinking structures were damaged. She could no longer identify or classify people in present time. Mike, the music therapist, looked like her lover. Mike became her lover. People from the past often replace people in the present in very old age. Pent-up rage finally splattered into the open. Millie could not control her feelings, and she didn't want to.

Before she died, Millie needed to express her hurt and pain. In the final Resolution Struggle, she wanted to heal herself. She needed someone to acknowledge her emotions, to validate her. But, no one did.

The validating worker knows that Millie's behavior in very old age is not psychotic or mindless. Millie was never mentally ill. She always functioned.

Here is the scene replayed with Validation.

Millie: "BITCH! Get me the hell outta' here."

Katie: (catching the fury in Millie's voice, reflecting her anger, using Rephrasing) "You hate this place!"

Millie: "Damn right. And everybody in it."

Katie: (using Polarity) "What do you hate the most?"

Millie: (curling her upper lip, leering, her voice high-pitched) "You."

Katie: (using Factual Language, exploring facts with questions) "What bothers you about me?"

Millie: "Your baby blue eyes, all decked out, ready to snatch all the men. There's a word for you. I'll spell it: W-O-R—whore."

Wanting to laugh at Millie's misspelling, Katie Centers. Laughing would have ruined their relationship. Katie is beginning to build trust. Millie's eyes no longer squint. Her voice is less harsh. Her chin no longer sticks out. Her facial muscles are more relaxed. Her breathing is more even.

Katie: (rephrasing) "Are you saying that I put on too much eye make-up to attract men?"

Millie: "And you're a whore. I see you making eyes at Harold; don't think I don't know what you're after."

Katie: (using a vague pronoun, "he," to replace "Harold" and "her" for someone in Millie's past.) "Did he leave you for her?"

Millie: (spitting on the floor) "The son of a bitch! He never wrote. He never called. I HATE HIM!"

Katie: "He really led you on?"

Millie: (her eyes watering, lower lip quivering, hurt reflected deep in her eyes) "What do you think?"

Katie: (softly) "You never saw him again?"

Millie: (in a whisper) "I saw him 25 years later with his wife and son across the street. He never saw me."

Katie: (gently stroking Millie's shoulder) "You never could love anyone else?"

Millie: (sobbing, her arms around Katie) "He was my whole life. I hate him."

Katie holds Millie until her sobs subside. The two women share an intimate moment. Millie feels validated, her grief and hurt ventilated. Her self-respect is returned. Katie feels the joy of communicating humanely and effectively with another human being.

A REMINISCING GROUP OR
A VALIDATION GROUP? WHAT IS THE DIFFERENCE?

Reminiscing—effective with a group of oriented or Maloriented very old people—can cause disaster with those who are in Time Confusion or Repetitive Motion. Laura Thomas misplaced words. Often, but not always, she smeared similar sounds together, creating her unique vocabulary. She no longer knew where she was. She had lost clock time, wavering between Time Confusion and Repetitive Motion.

GET HER OUTTA' HERE

Sally, an activity worker hoping to preserve Laura Thomas' speech, invited Laura to join the newly formed Reminiscing group. Here, residents could share pleasant past memories.

The topic for the day: "How did you celebrate Thanksgiving?" Six women and two men, ranging from 86 to 94 years, sat in a circle, not looking at each other. Sally wheeled in Mrs. Thomas and introduced her to the group.

"Her shoe squeaks," Mrs. Arvey's whiny voice pierced the silence. Ninety-three years old, she drooped, hunched in her wheelchair, her blurry blue eyes scanning the floor. The group ignored her. Mrs. Arvey was verbal, but she had lost her social controls. She swept the floor with her big toe in a grand gesture, waving a bony forefinger at Laura Thomas. "Get her outta' here."

Sally, in a low voice gently admonished, "Mrs. Thomas is going to join our group. Why don't we seat her right here? Sally placed Laura Thomas' wheelchair next to one of the men whose eyes were closed and whose chin wavered precariously, drifting lower and lower. "Today, we want to find out what you did on Thanksgiving." Sally's voice was cheery, full of energy. Silence sifted through the room. "Mr. Jones," Sally addressed a good-looking man of 87, with bright brown eyes. "You were born in New York City. How did you spend Thanksgiving? Did your mother make a turkey?"

Harry Jones smiled at Sally, his false teeth clacking in preparation for speech. "I can't hear you, sweetheart. You're sitting too far away. Why don't you come over and sit on my lap?" He chuckled and leered.

Sally swallowed her embarrassment and turned to Tessie Lew, the most oriented group member. "Mrs. Lew, you were born in New York, too. Can you tell us, in a loud voice so that Mr. Jones can hear, how you celebrated Thanksgiving?"

Mrs. Lew, age 89, had jet-black hair, streaked with grey patches, tied in a bun. Her wide forehead furrowed into hundreds of teeny wavy lines.

"I'm afraid," she started in a high, squeaky voice, "I can't talk loud, but I can tell you all that our Thanksgiving was the best ever. My mother made a turkey with all the trimmings. I have her recipe. I learned it by heart....."

"Shut up, slut. I don't give a damn about your mother and her turkey." Mr. Jones' husky voice drowned Mrs. Lew's recipe. Undaunted, she continued. Laura Thomas, rose from her wheelchair, wobbling, crying, silencing the duet: "I have to go home. My mother is waiting. I must treeple the sinomats before Dad sees them." She jerked her body forward, pulling at the arms of the chair that stifled her movements.

"But, Mrs. Thomas," Sally cried, replacing the old woman's body in the chair, "you'll fall if you walk. Please tell us about your Thanksgiving."

"Let me out. I have to go home. Hellpen. Healpen."

Sally called for help. The meeting was over.

These old nursing home residents could not function in a verbal Reminiscing group. Their attention span was too short; their logical, verbal skills too meager to respond to one topic. They could not separate past from present time, so they could not reminisce. They no longer had the words. They had lost social skills, moving on an emotional, not on a verbal, logical level.

Verbal, oriented residents who can remember the past, such as Mrs. Lew, flourish in a Reminiscing group. Here they can restore their identity and gain feelings of worth.

In a Validation group, where the topic is not thought provoking, but emotional, group members can relate to each other. When Mr. Jones asks the worker to sit on his lap, he is not ignored. The worker asks: "You miss your wife, don't you, Mr. Jones? Did she sit on your lap?" The Validation worker tunes into the old man's emotional needs. He always had good sex with his wife. His desire remains, even at age 87. The validating worker helps the group share common needs by expressing emotions through words, movement, and music.

"You betcha.' C'mon over, sweetheart." Harry Jones winks broadly.

The Validation worker makes close, intimate eye contact with this old man, asking: "Did you love her a lot?"

"Damn right." The old man's eyes gleam.

"Should we sing 'Let Me Call You Sweetheart' in honor of Mr. Jones wife? Mrs. Lew, can you be our song leader and start us out? Can we hold hands to feel close to each other. Mr. Jones, can you hold Mrs. Thomas' hand? I think she misses her husband, too."

The Validation worker knows each group member well. Mrs. Lew was a kindergarten teacher and loves her role as song leader. The group sings with gusto. The theme is "Missing Your Loved One." Group members look at each other. They express their longing. Music and movement bring them close.

PSYCHOTHERAPY

Psychotherapy involves a verbal relationship between a client and a therapist. Through this special relationship, the client reveals important feelings and facts about his or her life. The goal of psychotherapy is insight, a combination of intellectual and emotional awareness that enables people to understand their unhealthy living patterns and defense mechanisms and change their behaviors. Through psychotherapy, more positive coping methods are identified and more meaningful relationships with other people are established.

Validation and psychotherapy share certain basic beliefs. Both hold that people suffer when they suppress negative emotions and feel better when they express their emotions to a trusted listener. Both believe that early patterns of coping affect behavior throughout one's life and that people can change their behavior only when they want to do so. Both seek to raise self-esteem in order to increase the sense of well-being and ability to cope with stress.

Because of the very nature of psychotherapy, however, it is not appropriate for people in Resolution. Maloriented people do not want insight. They become hostile and anxious and blame, whine, or withdraw if they are confronted with their emotions. People in Resolution have spent lifetimes denying their feelings, and cannot find new ways of coping with these feelings in old age. Instead, they cling to well-established living patterns. Denial is their only way of surviving the stresses of daily life. Validation accepts the behavior of people in Resolution and does not try to change their ways of coping by providing them with insight. Instead, the validating caregiver listens empathetically to the negative emotions expressed by these people.

People in Time Confusion or Repetitive Motion are unable to benefit from psychotherapy because they have lost the ability to reflect. Moreover, they are unable to communicate verbally. Validation accepts their intellectual and physical deterioration and respects their nonlogical, intuitive wisdom. It uses verbal and nonverbal techniques to create an intimate relationship with an old-old person in order to restore the feeling of well-being.

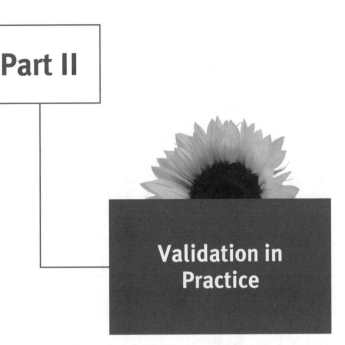

Part II

Validation in Practice

Part II presents very old people in different stages of Resolution in long-term care facilities, in a hospital, in senior housing, and in their own homes. Chapter 10 introduces five Maloriented people; Chapter 11 sketches three Time Confused people; Chapter 12 describes two Repetitive Movers. These chapters—based on vivid composites of real people with whom I have worked—show how the Validation techniques presented in Chapter 2 are used in real-life situations. All three of these chapters show how nurses, a doctor, community workers, nursing assistants, social workers, and family members learn to ease their frustration and help the very old person through Validation.

Chapter 13 follows the struggle of three very old Maloriented and Time Confused people to survive in the community. In 2000, 10 million Americans were over 65 years old. One third of these people had some form of dementia. Our hospitals and nursing homes were overflowing. In the upcoming years as these numbers continue to grow, we will be forced to help the old-old stay in their own homes as long as possible. More and more of us will meet Maloriented and disoriented very old people. More and more of us will have to learn how to communicate with them. What do we do with an 82-year-old man who can no longer find his way to the drug store and blames his neighbor for changing the street signs? How do we deal with an 85-year-old woman who absentmindedly drops her Social Security checks into the garbage and accuses the mailman of losing her mail? The graphic vignettes in Chapter 13 illustrate how ordinary people—a mailman, a grocery clerk, a hairdresser, an emergency medical technician—use Validation to help their old-old neighbors maintain dignity and independence. Chapter 14 discusses Validation for family members.

Chapter 10

Communicating with People Who Are Maloriented

ELLEN, THE HOARDER:
"WHEN YOU LISTEN, I SPEAK CLEAR"

Thick lashes lifted to reveal angry brown eyes. Ellen Haskins bolted toward me, bouncing her walker, meeting me head-on, outside of the doorway of The Home. It was 8:30 A.M. She was waiting to greet me with a sneer, curling her lips. "Hotsy totsy social worker with a master's degree. Ha! You're a master of dummies. You think you know everything, but you didn't know *that*, did you?" We walked inside to the dining room. In a grand gesture, her hand swept over the heads of 83 old people having breakfast. "Look at these dummies! They give me a pain in the neck!" Her chin, dotted with tiny white whiskers, jutted out, and her

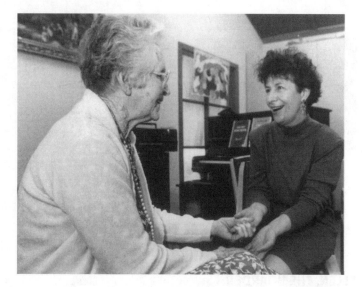

eyes narrowed in disgust. She reached for a wrought iron wastebasket. "Look at this!"

She dumped the contents, turning the wastebasket upside-down, littering the tile floor. She picked up a gold band hidden inside a banana peel. Gently, she wiped away the debris, producing a shiny wedding ring, which she shook under my nose. "Now, that is a disgrace. The last thing my husband said before he died was, 'Ellen, never take your wedding ring off your finger!' Do you see it on my finger? No. Where was my ring? In the trash! How did it get there? Huh? How?" I opened my mouth to answer. She shut it with, "I'll tell you how! They stole it. In the middle of the night, while I was fast asleep, they snuck into the room and stole my wedding ring. I'm not a sound sleeper. They're clever. They give out sleeping pills to knock people out so they can rob them at night."

In 2 years, Ellen Haskins had burnt us all out with her "paranoid" behavior. We did not "buy into her delusion" or "feed her fantasy." Day in and day out, Ellen would stash her gold band in the bottom of the wastebasket and then insist that someone had stolen it. We tried to change the subject when Ellen would begin to accuse. Finally, we avoided her altogether. Having spent too much energy on Ellen Haskins, we had given up trying to convince her. She herself had put her ring in the trash. The cleaning woman saw Ellen carefully stashing her gold band in the bottom of a wastebasket.

Her daughter flinched, red-faced with embarrassment, when Ellen accused her of stealing the ring. Ellen's voice would become mean, hateful, full of venom. "Don't you tell me that I put my own wedding ring in the trash! You think I'm crazy?" Ellen hurt the people she loved. She had no friends. Residents and staff called her "the bitch."

In 1975, the psychiatrist diagnosed her as "paranoid, with delusions of persecution." In 1979, after a CT scan, the neurologist ruled out reversible conditions, such as subdural hematoma. His diagnosis was "probable Alzheimer's disease, late-onset dementia." Her test results showed failure in four spheres: 1) memory, 2) judgment, 3) problem-solving performance, and 4) ability to perform in the community. Her personal care functions were found to be unimpaired. A physical examination found her to be a fairly healthy, normal 86-year-old female, with some osteoarthritis and no reversible conditions that might account for her dementia.

Ellen's speech was clear and her remote memory intact. She would forget names, but kept careful track of present time and place. If I was 3 minutes late for our appointment, her foot would tap impatiently marking the time, as she greeted me with "Do you know what time it is?"

Occasionally, Ellen would forget the name of The Home, something that would cause her to panic. Terrified of falling apart, Ellen used filler words to cover. Her voice would become shrill, her words tumbled. "Of course I know the name of this place. You think I'm crazy? Haven't I lived here for years? Why do you keep asking me so many stupid questions? Don't you have better things to do?"

Ellen Haskins was 85 years old when she began accusing people of dumping her wedding ring in the trash. She had led a productive life and had no history of mental illness. After her first husband died in World War I, Ellen struggled as a bookkeeper to raise her three children, succeeding in sending all of them to college. Her daughter told me that Ellen had been a strict parent, never expressing her love. "We were not a touchy-feely family," she told me. Ellen Haskins held herself erect, often reporting with pride, "I taught my children how to be neat. Everything in its proper place. Socks have to be folded just so! My mother was a very clean person, God rest her soul. We didn't dare mess up. I brought up my children the same way." At age 46, Ellen Haskins fell in love and remarried. Two years later, her second husband died of a heart attack while they were hiking. Ellen went back to work.

At age 86, Ellen's body was a summary of how she had led her life. Bold, direct eye contact; neck muscles tight; chin jutted out; movements precise; speech crisp and clear. She often complained of a pain in her neck. Her favorite phrase: "Life is a pain in the neck!" She was a "no-nonsense" person. She held on. She did not want to be touched. She did not express emotions.

Ellen was afraid of losing control. To keep herself together, she hoarded. Newspapers she had saved for 20 years lined her drawers and covered every inch of floor under her bed. When the cleaning women wanted to sweep under her bed, Ellen stopped them. Arms folded, her voice level, Ellen would order them to leave. "Get out of my room, and leave my things alone. Those papers belong there." Her purse, filled with faded newspaper clippings from World War I, was tucked under her arm and went with her everywhere.

Ellen was struggling to tie up loose ends in the Resolution Stage of life. Unconsciously, she longed to put her life in order. She had never properly expressed fury or grief when she lost one husband and then another. When she lost the men she loved, life had dumped her, like her ring, into the trash can. Now I found her using her wedding ring to express her deep sorrow and helpless resentment.

Ellen Haskins taught me the first principle of Validation—build trust by accepting feelings; don't argue the facts. Ellen was using her wedding ring indirectly to express her feelings of being dumped, feelings that she was afraid to express directly. For 60 years, she had accumulated unresolved emotions. To unleash her suppressed anger at losing her husbands, she hid her wedding ring so that she could accuse the world of robbing her. The wedding ring symbolized her lost loves. She could not express her anger and grief directly, so she used her wedding ring. The Validation worker does not call this behavior paranoid, because this was her only way of expressing her deep loss. Her blaming and accusing helped heal her hurt. She needed someone to listen. Then her blaming would lessen. She had to hold onto familiar patterns. Arguing with her or reorienting her to the facts made her worse. Blaming was a way of coping. Ignored like Isadore Rose, she would have withdrawn inward.

Blamers are mean old men and women. Ellen Haskin's daughter, Mary, learned to Center in order to wash away her hurt when her mother began to blame. To validate her mother, Mary had to acknowledge her hurt, put it in the closet, close the door, and listen with empathy. It is harder for a family member than for a professional to validate the blamer. Emotions get in the way. The hurt is greater. Mary wanted her mother to be the same vital "normal" person she knew as a girl. Now, the kinder Mary was, the more her mother blamed. "Why is Mother so mean?" Mary often cried. The closer the relationship, the harder it is to listen without judging. Validation requires genuine, open, nonjudgmental listening—empathy. Sometimes, the Maloriented old person will provoke feelings of anger, outrage, humor, or pain in the caregiver. The caregiver Centers. When Mary put her feelings in the closet, she was able to listen with an open mind. Her voice held respect, despite Ellen's outrageous behavior. Even if deaf, the Maloriented old person will "hear" the listener's impatient sigh; even if blind, the old person will "see" the frustrated frown of the listener. Mary learned to listen exquisitely, becoming free to hear the undertones in her mother's voice. For a son or daughter, this is not easy. Centering helps!

Blamers are afraid of feelings. When I tried to soothe Ellen by saying, "That must make you feel terrible," she glared at me, and responded in a biting voice, "I feel fine. There is nothing to talk about!" Instead of patronizing Ellen, I learned to walk beside her, respecting her space. I learned not to divert her or placate her, not to ask her to expose her feelings or to figure out why she behaved the way she did. Ellen did not want to understand her own behavior. When I gave up trying to change her, when I stopped trying to give her insight, she began to trust me.

"What was your first husband like? How old were you when he gave you the wedding ring?" I asked Ellen.

Her eyes softened as she recalled. "Harry gave me the ring when I was 16. We found it in an old jewelry store on 14th Street."

I listened without interrupting. I never probed. Ellen was healing herself in her own way, by talking about her husband. Her feelings of love and pain came out as she remembered his death. She had lost the angry look in her eyes, her breathing became more even. Her facial muscles relaxed, her voice softened.

When Ellen accused the cleaning lady of hiding her ring, I didn't argue. I listened without judging, using nonthreatening factual words to explore. "*When* did she steal your ring, Mrs. Haskins?" I asked.

Recognizing the sincerity in my voice, Ellen did a double take. "That awful woman comes in the middle of the night, when I'm sound asleep. They're smart, those people. They take advantage of you when you're not looking, when you least expect it. That's when they rob you."

In spitting out her anger at the staff, Ellen was getting rid of pent-up rage against the world. Her fury, expressed at last and acknowledged by someone she was beginning to trust, began to melt. Her blaming lessened. Others noticed the change in Ellen's behavior. I taught Laura, the wise housekeeper who cleaned Ellen's room, the first two steps of Validation. Laura, her face crinkled with caring, listened closely. She understood. She quickly learned how to Center and to validate Ellen.

"Laura, I had 10 oranges in my sink. There are only three left. You know I keep them there to refrigerate them. You had no business removing my property. You stole my oranges. Put them right back!" said Ellen one morning.

Instead of angrily denying the charge of stealing Ellen's fruit, Laura responded with a tone of respect. "How many oranges did you have, Mrs. Haskins?"

"You heard me. There were 10 oranges in that sink. My daughter mailed them to me from Florida."

Laura continued to validate Ellen. "Your daughter thinks about you even when she's on a vacation! What kind of oranges were they?"

"They were Sunkist," answered Ellen, "and only grown for export. You can't even buy them in Florida."

"Your daughter knows how to shop," said Laura. "How did you bring her up?"

"I had to teach her. You know, we lived through the Depression. We couldn't afford oranges, and I loved them so. My mother always gave me oranges for my birthday. Big, juicy ones," said Ellen, her anger already diminishing.

"What was it like during the Depression?" asked Laura.

"We didn't even have an icebox that worked right," whined Ellen.

"It must have been tough bringing up children then," Laura responded.

"Would you have liked to live like that? I had to wipe them with newspapers. We couldn't even afford toilet paper. Sometimes their little behinds would bleed, poor things."

Ellen and Laura continued to talk for another 5 minutes, sharing experiences, trusting each other. Laura understood that Ellen Haskins had grown up hoarding in order to keep herself together. Ellen felt safe when she had her possessions in one place. As a child, she had learned to put the right thing in the right place at the right time in order to be loved. In her old age, Ellen Haskins had lost her home, her husbands. The more she lost, the more she held on. During the Depression, she ran out of money. Now, she was running out of family and friends, out of her role in life. Her hoarding got worse.

Bottled-up feelings of loss had festered inside Ellen for a lifetime. She would never expose feelings directly. Her anger and fear were carefully disguised. She used oranges, her wedding ring, tiny bits of tissue carefully folded in triangles, to express her fear and maintain her control. As we listened to the facts, never arguing, Ellen's fury lost its strength. Although disguised, her feelings were exposed to the light of day. We spent 5 minutes, each day, listening to Ellen. Within months, she stopped accusing staff or her daughter of stealing her wedding ring.

LUCY, THE SPITTER: "BITCH! GET OUT OF MY ROOM!"

Lucy Kelly spat. She often spat at people she didn't like, and Lucy did not like me. Her voice grumbled, deep in her throat. "Goddamn son of a bitch, get the hell outta' my room. Bitch!"

The last "bitch" was punctuated by spit, which hit the mark. I blinked.

"Well, aren't you gone yet?" Lucy accentuated her words by jabbing me with the tip of her cane.

With some effort, I shut out the anger and kept my voice calm. Patiently, I reasoned with her. "Mrs. Kelly, my job is to help you feel better."

She mimicked the tone of my voice to ridicule me. "I don't want to feel better, so you better find another job. I don't talk to idiots."

"I like my job, and I like you," I said feebly. "I want to help you."

"LIAR!" she shrieked.

Lucy spoke the truth. I could not like her. Her beady brown eyes shot out hate. Her cheeks, swollen with medications, puffed in and out like an accordion. I stared at her for a moment, then softly said goodbye.

In the hallway, I began to cry, without knowing why. As a professional social worker trained to understand and accept all human behaviors, I should not have reacted emotionally.

The next day, I tried to give Lucy insight. I wanted her to understand why she was so full of hate, to become aware of the reasons behind her fury, to want to change her behaviors. She was lying stiff as a board, her back rigid, her face turned to the wall. Tentatively, I approached her bed. "Mrs. Kelly, it's me, Naomi. Are you still angry?" I waited but there was no answer. In desperation, I continued exploring her feelings, trying to build a relationship. "I don't blame you for feeling angry, Mrs. Kelly. You have lots of reasons. I know how you feel. You were an active woman. Now, you can't even walk." Lucy Kelly remained silent. I gulped and went on in a shaky voice. "You've lost your wonderful job, your husband, and your friends. People looked up to you. You were the life of the party. No wonder you're angry at the world. I would feel angry too."

"Oh, shut up, you fool! I don't care how you feel. You can jump out the window as far as I care. AND DON'T TELL ME HOW I FEEL! I AM NOT ANGRY. NOW GET THE HELL OUT OF MY ROOM BEFORE I CALL SOMEONE TO DRAG YOU OUT! DON'T YOU KNOW WHEN YOU'RE NOT WANTED?" Her voice became cold and mean. Clearly, Lucy did not want to get in touch with her feelings. Like Ellen Haskins and Isadore Rose, she did not want to know why she was so angry. She did not want to change. She could not trust herself or others. Since facing her fears might mean losing control, Lucy denied feelings. I was not about to change her at this stage in her life, when her world had fallen apart.

Lucy Kelly had been a successful businesswoman, the head buyer for a large department store. Her daughter, Norma, told me that she had always been bossy. "When

Mother opened her mouth, everyone listened and did just what she said. She would tell Dad that I was naughty and Dad would punish me without asking me what had happened. Mother was always right." Lucy's daughter's voice trembled. "When my mother calls me, my heart lurches. To this day, I jump. And I am 54 years old!" The daughter's blue eyes blinked hard with held-back tears. "When I was 10, I forgot to cross a 'T' on my homework essay. Mother made me write and rewrite the paragraph, smacking my hand when my letters weren't perfectly even. My tears splashed onto the ink and blurred the words. I never did hand in that essay and got a detention. Dad punished me hard. I'll never forget hating my mother that night." Norma, Lucy's daughter, ended in a soft, apologetic voice, wanting to control the flood of memory.

Norma read the empathy in my eyes, and we both felt better. I suddenly experienced my own flashback. I had hated playing the piano, but my mother made me take piano lessons. My turn came at the big recital. I froze and sat there like a dumbbell. Mother got up; gave me an icy, unforgiving stare; and stalked out of the hall, with 85 people watching.

A big chunk, like a brick of ice, worked on my heart. Something heavy inside struggled to come out. I had to face my anger at my mother or carry the burden of hate to my old age. Would I end up alone? Like Lucy Kelly—self-centered, bitter, blaming, full of self-hate and hate for others? Would I alienate my children? If we stay frozen in the past, we might become stuck in anger at age 85.

Norma wondered at my sudden silence. I needed to teach her to face her hate so that she could move on. I spoke slowly, the words forming themselves with care. "Your mother hurt you terribly, and you hated her. Feel that hate!"

Norma stared for a moment. Her face lit with awareness. "My mother is a bitch!"

I nodded. "Can you forgive her?"

Norma smiled wryly, her feelings relieved. "Naomi, if you help me, I'll give it my best shot. I don't want to become like her when I get old."

Once we had faced the hurt and the hate, Norma and I could Center, wash away our own feelings, closet them, and tune into Lucy's world. From Lucy, I learned that we cannot help blamers unless we first acknowledge our own anger and lay it aside. I was learning the importance of insight into my own hang-ups. I was preparing for my own wise old age—a dividend I earned through struggling to empathize with Lucy. I tried different ways of building trust. I learned Validation the hard way. I made mistakes.

"Good morning, Mrs. Kelly," my voice sang, bouncing with cheer.

"Oh, shut up. What's good about it?" Lucy's voice was dull and flat. She spoke to the wall.

I echoed her voice tone, rephrasing her words, "Are you saying that there is nothing good about the morning?"

"That's right, you said it," she answered.

She was talking to me. Her face turned slightly in my direction. I continued paraphrasing her words, reflecting her attitude with respect. "You wake up and nothing matters anymore, is that it?," I asked.

"That's it. That's the way it is—no more, no less. So why don't you leave me alone. Scat!" She shot out the words, only half meaning them. There was a pleading undertone to her words.

Encouraged, I continued rephrasing. "With nothing to do, there's no use in talking?" I ended with a question in my voice to be sure that I had understood her meaning.

Lucy sat upright in her bed. "You said it!" She looked me straight in the eye for the first time. Our relationship had begun. Just rephrasing her words had worked.

Lucy Kelly had taught me Validation Technique 3: rephrase the person's words and reflect the person's attitude without judgment or analysis—how simple! Matching Lucy's voice-tone was harder. Feelings would creep into my voice. With the sensitivity of a Geiger counter, Lucy could detect even the tiniest false note. Like a turtle, she would then retreat and withdraw inside her shell. To reflect her tone honestly, I had to keep myself Centered. Five to ten respectful, genuine minutes with Lucy was all I could manage once a day.

Once we began to communicate, I used Validation Technique 2: exploring with factual questions. "Mrs. Kelly," I would ask, "what does a buyer in a big department store do?"

"Too much—I was busy from the minute I got up to the minute I went to bed." Her voice held pride. For Lucy, work was everything. Out of a job, she was nothing. With nobody to boss, she felt helpless. She didn't know how to act when the losses hit.

In the weeks to come, Lucy and I spent quality time every day remembering her busy life. She never learned to understand why she held onto worn out roles, why she stagnated in her old age. But Lucy did not withdraw inward. She spoke to her daughter more civilly.

Lucy's daughter, Norma, also learned to validate Lucy. It was not easy. Lucy had become a cruel person in her old age, and her cruelty extended even to her great-grandchildren. One day Norma brought her granddaughter to visit Lucy. "Look, Mother, here's Susy. Aren't you going to open your eyes and say hello to your great-grandchild?"

Lucy remained silent. Norma pleaded. "Please, Mother, open your eyes."

Lucy slowly lifted half a lid of one cataract-blurred eye. "Very nice. Now let me go back to sleep." Her low, gruff voice cut like a knife. She closed both eyes tight and turned her back.

"Mother, you made me feel bad." Norma was hurt by her mother's selfishness. Lucy snorted, her voice muffled by the wall.

"Don't you care about your great-granddaughter? About me?" Norma cried.

Lucy snorted, "I want to get out of here. I want to walk out. I want to get back to my job. If you do that for me, I'll talk to your family."

"Mother, they are your family, too. Don't you love us?" cried Norma.

Lucy snorted again. Her back stayed stiff. "If you loved me, you'd help me get out of this place and back to work."

"Mother, you need medications. I can't lift you. You can't bend your knees. How can you get up and go back to work?" asked Norma... No answer. Norma tried again, stuffing down her irritation. Her voice edgy, Norma leaned over to look at her mother, "Mother, please, be reasonable. I can't do what you want. I know you hate it here, but there's nothing I can do."

"If you cared, you'd do something. You don't care." Lucy began to spit.

Norma Centered herself. Facing her frustration helped her lay aside her simmering resentment. Then she spoke quietly, rephrasing with empathy, "Mother, you think that if I cared about you, I would take you out of here?"

Surprised at the quiet, caring tone, Lucy nodded. "That's right. I'm a burden to you. You don't want me around."

Again, Norma rephrased. "You think that nobody wants to be with you because you can't walk or work?"

"That's exactly what I think. Without my legs and my job, I might as well be dead." Lucy's voice lost some of its bitterness and took on some longing. "Dad felt the same way when he couldn't walk, Norma," Lucy's voice dropped. "Dad was miserable. He was so ashamed when he couldn't even wipe himself. He was a proud man." Lucy began to cry.

"Mother," Norma said gently, "it's hard for you, too, isn't it?"

Lucy nodded bitterly. "I worked all my life, Norma. Now, I'm useless. I can't stand it. I wish I were dead, like Dad. He suffered terribly. I heard him cry when he thought nobody was listening." Lucy's voice sobered at the painful memory.

"Did Dad ever get used to being paralyzed?" Norma and Lucy remembered together. Each day they built a relationship.

Norma no longer tried to calm her mother down. She accepted Lucy the way she was, and validated her mother's feelings without judging. This is not easy for an adult child who longs for a wise, dignified mother to love, a mother who deals with the losses of old age without hitting back at her children. This kind of mother is a rare gift. I hope that I will be giving that gift to my children when my strength fails and I need their help.

SADIE, THE MARTYR: "ONE MOTHER HAS TEN KIDS. TEN KIDS CAN'T CARE FOR ONE MOTHER!"

"Ma, you used a bad word!" Eight-year-old Kenny's eyes sparkled with mischievous glee. He didn't notice his mother's hands twisting the telephone receiver she was holding away from her ear. He only heard the "bad" word and wondered how his mother was going to worm herself out of his trap.

"Honey, sometimes there is no other word. You only use that word when you are desperate—in an emergency. Do you understand?" Marge bent down to look straight into her son's wide open brown eyes. A moment between them clicked.

The little boy nodded briefly and ran out to play, yelling to his mother over his shoulder, "Yeah, Mom! Bye!" The screen door slammed.

Marge smiled, a grin of gratitude for having a wise son. Then she stiffened, returning to the telephone. Her thin fingers shuffled through her prematurely greying hair. She pulled out one white hair and threw it in the garbage, praying, "Dear God, please help me never, never to act like my mother when I get old. Please let me die first!"

Marge's voice began pleading. "Mother, we've talked for 55 minutes. Thank God the baby's still asleep. I can't leave my family and take the next plane to Indianapolis. You've got four children who live 30 minutes from your house. Can't you call Lillian or Joan? Mother...don't cry...please, Mother...I love you. I don't want you to be miserable all the time. Mother, what's the matter? What happened?"

Marge heard her mother gasp for breath. Then silence. Marge screamed into the telephone. "Mother! What's the matter? Should I call an ambulance?"

Her mother's voice came through clear and strong. "Margaret, I have to dial 911."

Marge's mother, Sadie, hung up. Marge stared at the dead receiver and replaced the telephone. Without pity it rang again. Marge jumped, unprepared for the second shrill, relentless ring. Sighing, she replaced anger with resignation and picked up the receiver. Her mother's voice was frantic. "911 is busy. What should I do? Tell me! Quick, before it's too late. I can't breathe. My breath is gone. Hear it? Like a sheet of metal around my heart, squeezing my breath away. This is the end. Oh! It hurts so bad. It's spreading to my back. It's choking me."

Marge heard raspy spurts of air quickening over the phone. "Mother, close your mouth. That's right. Breathe slowly through your nose—in through your nose and out of your mouth. Take deep breaths. Rest your hands on your stomach. That's right... good... that sounds much better. Keep breathing that way... don't stop. Turn on the television. Watch and breathe for 5 minutes. I'll call Lillian and Joan, and we'll decide what to do."

Marge had been through this scene a hundred times in the past 6 months. A Validation therapist had taught Marge how to Center and wash away her anger. When Marge's father died 2 years ago, her mother had collapsed. After the funeral service, Sadie had moaned to her children, "Daddy is dead, and you should now bury me. After 44 years, I'm alone. Harry!" Sadie's eyes lifted to heaven, imploring the clouds that drifted nonchalantly by, ignoring her. She raised both arms in prayer: "Take me! I'm 72 years old. I've lived a good life. I've raised 10 children. They have good jobs. They have families. They're busy people. They can't afford to spend time with an old woman who is all alone. I had time for them. Please, God. If you have a heart, take me." Sadie rocked back and forth in anguish, eyes shut tight, squeezing out a tear or two.

"Mother, we'll take you. You can live with us. We have room, now that Chuck is married." Sadie's eldest daughter made the offer, gladly. Her husband nodded.

Sadie had been a devoted mother. Her children had been her life. She had sacrificed an acting career to have a family. If not for her five children, Sadie would have become a Broadway star, without a doubt. Six famous directors had told her so. Her adoring husband believed her story. Each one of Sadie's children had been nursed on that story. They believed it. Sadie believed it.

Sadie slowly lowered her eyes from heaven and returned to her children. Her eyes calm, subdued, in dulcet tones, she demurred, "No, thank you very much, but no. I have my own house, where I lived with my husband . . ." her voice broke. Sadie swallowed to gain control and continued, ". . . for over 44 years. The same house with the same man for over 44 years. How can I move? Even to a child's house? It's too late to make a change. I'll scrape together what money I have left. I'll manage. I'll be fine." Sadie's children respected her strength and left her alone.

Sadie mourned for 1 year. Newspapers found their way to the trash, unread. Dishes piled up. Shades stayed down. Sadie shut out the traffic of the world. Her children ached for her. They took her shopping. They bought her groceries. They urged her to live with them. Staunchly, with pride, Sadie refused.

One year and 6 months after her husband died, Sadie began her "organ recitals." She started small, but with practice she honed her skill. She would usually begin with the top of her body and move down. Her organ recitals had a beginning, a middle, and a grand finale. "My head hurts. Oh! What a headache. Aspirins don't help. If you could only feel the pounding—like a sledgehammer on my temples. This time, it hits my heart. Don't tell me it's heartburn. I never had heartburn in my life. I know heartburn from heart failure—a dull pain that grips you, squeezing you, cutting your heart out. Your grandmother died from congestive heart failure. So did your Uncle Jake. He walked in the door one night ... Woop ... Two minutes ... hello, goodbye, he was gone. Dropped dead on the front porch—right there, on the third step. Honey, rub my lower back. I can't move. It's a sharp pain. I'm paralyzed. Help me, Honey. How can I get to the bathroom?" Sadie's voice drops to a whisper, "and when I get there, *nothing comes out.*" Sadie looks around, dumbfounded. "I was never constipated in my whole life. My bowels were perfect—regular as clockwork, once a day. Now, I'm lucky if I can go once a week. Maybe it's *cancer of the colon.* That's the worst cancer—the colon. The most painful. Oh! it hurts all over." The finale was dialing 911.

Marge had listened to this recital for too long. The slam of the screen door broke her reflection. "Mom, I want a sandwich," Kenny said, rummaging through the refrigerator, spilling a half-filled glass of milk.

"Kenny! Look at the mess you've made. How can you do that? Don't you have any sense?" Marge shrieked, her voice cracking with strain.

"Mother, you're getting hyper. Cool it." Kenny wiped up the spilt milk, shrugging his shoulders.

Marge's guilt struck her like a knife. I'm taking out my anger at my mother by yelling at my son, she thought. I've got to handle it better. Marge took Ken's hand and softly admitted, "Ken, I'm worried about Grandma. I'm sorry if I've been taking it out on you."

"It's okay, Mom. But you better fix it up before you explode." Kenny ran from the room.

Marge nodded and took some deep breaths to Center when the telephone rang and her 18-month-old daughter started to cry at the same moment. Marge scooped up her baby and picked up the telephone.

"Margaret, I am sure that I'm dying. You have got to come out here right away. None of the other children understand what I'm going through. Margaret, do you hear me? I need you right now. You can't wait. If you wait it will be too late. I will be gone." Sadie's voice rose. She breathed hard into the telephone.

Marge felt rage blowing up inside her like a balloon. Sensing Marge's fury, the baby cried louder. Marge shouted into the receiver, her voice desperate and final. "Mother, I cannot leave my children and fly to Indianapolis. I just can't. You've got four other children to call. Call them!" Marge heard a click. Her mother had hung up. Her baby screaming, Marge called her four brothers and sisters. Each one had suffered similar telephone calls from Sadie. Each one had had it. Each one wanted to give up.

Marge called me next. In my office, she was jumpy, her eyes puffy with dried-up tears. She paced back and forth, stopping for a moment, pounding her knuckles to consider her next move.

"Should we place Mother in a nursing home? She's only 74 years old. I can't have her committed. And that's the only way we'd get her to a home. She would never leave her own home. She's said that a million times: 'I would rather die before going to a nursing home. Kill me first.'"

I tried to give Marge insight into her mother's typical way of dealing with hard times. "Marge, did your mother complain of aches and pains when you were growing up?"

Marge stopped pacing to remember. She thought hard. "When Dad lost his job, she got pneumonia. We had to live with our aunt for 6 months while Mother was in the hospital. When our grandmother died, Mother lost her voice. Her bronchial tubes closed, and they had to stick a tube down her throat so that she could breathe. I guess when things go wrong, Mother gets sick." Marge suddenly realized her mother's inability to face hard times. She began to empathize with her mother: the martyr.

"Marge, I've seen hundreds of martyrs. Their children want nothing to do with them. They lose their friends," I explain. "You love your mother. Maybe the Validation techniques will help."

"First, you need empathy. Find a time in your life when the bottom dropped out, when too much was going wrong at one time. That's how your mother feels now."

Marge bit her lower lip to remember. Her eyes lowered in pain. "When I had a miscarriage. The ache in the middle of my chest hurt most in the hospital when the nurse made her cheery, early morning announcement: 'Mothers, it's time to nurse your babies!' I could have slit her throat to shut her up." Marge's tears mingled with sad humor.

I said softly, "Marge, can you think of that ache when you listen to your mother?" She nodded.

I taught Marge how to explore by asking "who?" "what?" "where?" "when?" and "how?" She learned to rephrase her mother's complaints with *empathy.* Then, Marge learned Validation Technique 12: using the person's preferred sense.

"Marge, when your mother called you yesterday, what word did she use the most? Can you remember?"

Marge opened her eyes wide in wonder. "I had never considered that. Her favorite word is 'hurts'—this hurts, that hurts, it hurts all over. She could write a musical comedy, 'Oh! How Much It Hurts Me.'"

I smiled. "Then you use similar words. Speak her language. Step right into her world. Your mother seems to be mainly a feeling person. She prefers her sense of touch, her sensations. Use feeling words with her. Ask her how bad, or how sharp, or how dull the pain is. Is it the worst at night? Or during the day?"

Marge persisted, still unsure, "How long do these Validation sessions last? How do I end them? Do they go on forever?"

"Give her 5 exquisite minutes of listening. When her breathing slows down, her voice becomes less whiny, tell her you're sorry, but you have to hang up. You are a mother, responsible for young children. She'll understand that. But be sure to reassure her that you'll talk to her again soon. Don't forget when you promised to call her. Even if your kids get sick, remember to call her at *that time*. She'll count on you. Your Validation sessions need to go on until your mother dies. Martyrdom is your mother's Red Cross safety survival kit. She'll never go anywhere without it. She'll need a trusted listener to travel with, forever.

Six weeks later, telephone calls from Indianapolis sounded like this:

Sadie: *(her breath rising and falling like waves in a thunderstorm)* Come right away! I'm shaking all over.

Marge: Where are you shaking? In your hands?

Sadie: *(taking a moment to find out)* My hands? No. Not my hands? Yes. My hands. They are shaking so bad I can't even hold the telephone. It's dropping from my fingers.

Marge: Mother, try holding on for just one more minute. Take a deep breath. Where else in your body are you shaking?

Sadie: My heart. My heart is shaking... pounding... so hard ... *(Sadie's voice trails.)* my voice, too. Can't you hear how my voice is shaking?

Marge: I hear it. It's shaking so bad. Has it been shaking all day?

Sadie: Since this morning, when I got up. It started then. What shall I do?

Marge: Have you had breakfast yet?

Sadie: How can I eat when I can't even talk? When my voice is stuck in my throat? I can't find the words. I can't even swallow. There's a terrible lump in my throat.

Marge: *(Centering quickly, to restore her loving voice-tone)* There's a lump in your throat, Mother? What does the lump feel like? Does it hurt to swallow?

Sadie: It's too horrible to describe. The pain gets so bad I have to sit up in bed. I get up, I walk around, but nothing helps. I can't sleep a wink. *(Sadie's breathing quickens.)* Is this living? If this is living, dying is a gift from God.

Marge: Is it hard at night? Is that when you miss Dad the most? Is that when the pain feels the worst?

Sadie: *(now crying with relief)* Oh yes, honey. At night I miss Dad so much. It makes me shake all over when I think of being alone without him. That's when I get a lump in my throat. He was so good to me, Margaret. We lived together for such a long time. I can't bear to go on without him. *(Sadie's voice softens with longing.)*

Marge: Oh, Mother, it is so hard for you to stand so much pain. I wish I could be with you right now. Can you walk over to Joan's house and tell her how you feel? She needs to know how much Dad meant to you. She also needs help with her kids. You know how much Joan's kids love you.

Sadie went next door to Joan's. Marge was able to explain the Validation techniques to her sisters and brothers. Sadie never stopped her complaining, but there were many times when her organ recitals stopped sooner. More and more often the litany never even reached her stomach. She slept better at night. She died at age 81 in her own kitchen, a modified martyr.

PEG, THE WORRIER: "THERE'S A MAN UNDER MY BED!"

"I wish he wouldn't come tonight." Peg Harvey clunked her upper plate into the glass, enjoying the tinkling sound her teeth always made when she tucked them in for the night. She always brushed them the same way, quoting her mother: "Small, even, swift strokes to keep them white and pearly."

"Did you say you're getting up early?" Elsa, her roommate in the Hilltop Housing Development for the Elderly, shouted from her bed.

"Pearly, I said 'pearly,' not 'early.' Why don't you put on your hearing aid, Elsa? You never know what might happen during the night. At least you'll hear what they say about you before you go."

Elsa snapped, "I'm not going to die tonight. So shut up and let me go to sleep."

Peg, hurt at Elsa's cold voice-tone, whispered, "Well, I might die. Did you see the moon?" Peg peered at the silvery moon bobbing behind the clouds. "A full moon—I can tell. It's hiding its face in the clouds, but I know it's full. Elsa, did you hear me? THE MOON IS FULL!" Peg shouted.

Elsa jumped up and lashed out, "If you don't shut up and go to sleep, I'm going to call the Super, and they'll put you on the third floor in the 'D' building with the crazy people."

Afraid of the threat, Peg muttered under her breath, "She thinks I'm crazy, but wait until that man shows his

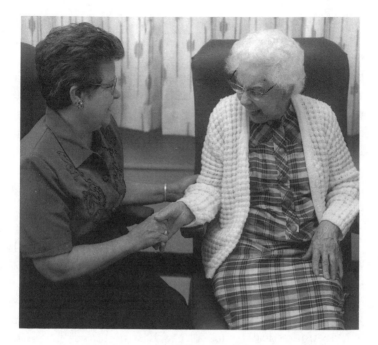

face to *her*. And God knows what else he'll show. Then, it'll be too late!" Cautiously, tentatively, Peg poked her big toe under her bed. Relieved, she waved her whole foot, feeling the space, whispering, "He's not there yet, but he's coming. I can smell it. Something has got to be done. When it's too late, they'll all believe me. God knows what he'll do to us. If only Peter would have waited one more year. Peter, why couldn't you wait to die? We would have had our insurance money, and I wouldn't have had to come to this place. It's easy for you. You're dead. I have to live with that Elsa who's almost stone deaf. Peter, listen to me. Tell me what to do. Should I go and tell the Super? He'll say I'm crazy. They'll put me in the other building on the third floor. That will be the end. The smell will kill me first. Second, I'll have to hear the crazy people yelling all day. No. But, I have to tell somebody. Shh, I think he's coming." Peg froze. Her skin, now covered with bristling goose-bumps, turned chalk white. She stopped breathing. She saw a form developing under her bed. First, the head, the neck, the shoulders, and then the rest of his body. It was a man, and he was naked. Peg fled from her room, her white nightgown ballooning, a sail in the wind, lifting her swiftly down the red carpeted hallway, through the lobby, and out into the moonlit night.

I saw Peg the next day. Primly, she sat apart from the other women, crocheting in the craft room. Her medical and social history told me that she had always been a relatively normal, albeit neurotic, woman. She had never been hospitalized for mental illness and was a physically healthy 82-year-old. Her two children lived far away, but cared about her, visiting at least twice a year. Last night was her fifth nocturnal episode. The administrator of the Senior Apartment complex was worried. Should Peg be moved to the Alzheimer's wing? Did she belong in a mental institution? Her mental status test results did not point to any form of dementia.

She smiled sweetly when I approached her, grateful for my attention. She looked sheepish when she saw me look around the room at the other women, who ignored us. Peg was obviously isolated. "The other ladies used to be my friends," she explained, apologetically. "Now, they don't want to sit near me because they know that I ran out of the building in the middle of the night. They all think I'm crazy." Peg blinked away a tear. She was hurt by the rejection. Her shoulders curved, her head burrowed in her chest, she would not look into my eyes.

Peg had the typical stance of the victim: shoulders rounded, eyes downcast, breathing slow, lips pursed, chin tucked in, movements indirect, body leaning forward. Victims walk slowly, bending low to protect themselves from the onslaught of humanity. They carry a heavy load. Emotionally, the victim is like the blamer. The victim does not face feelings. Like the blamer, in old age, the victim stays oriented to present time and place, but not happily. When victims survive to very old age, they become Maloriented, lugging their burden of suppressed emotions to the grave.

Peg hunched her shoulders, carrying the weight of the world on her back as we walked to my office. Sadly, she explained her slow gait. "I can't walk very fast because of my back. Lower back pain is very painful, so you'll have to bear with me. It's going to take awhile." I nodded. Peg wanted my time. She needed a friend. The tenants in her building walked away from her. They were afraid that her "hallucinations" would rub off on them. They were afraid of guilt by association. They were busy dealing with their own losses. They had no time left to listen to Peg's fears. Her ignored feelings were festering. Locked inside during the day, her fear gained strength at night.

Trying to change her behavior by ignoring it made it worse. Peg Harvey needed Validation. She needed someone to listen with care. In a respectful voice-tone, I applied Validation Technique 2: focusing on the factual.

"What happened last night, Mrs. Harvey?"

"Oh, it was terrible. He looked so evil." Peg's voice dropped in fear, her eyes looked up at the ceiling in vivid recall. When people look up, they often visualize something. I checked it out. "Mrs. Harvey, are you picturing him right now with your mind's eye?"

"Oh, yes. I see him clear as day, only he comes at night."

"What makes him come to you?"

Peg bit her lower lip in concentration. Her eyes stopped blinking, her forehead wrinkled in thought. She shook her head, "I don't know, but he only comes when there is a full moon. Last night, did you see it?" Peg didn't wait for me to answer, but rushed on. "A brilliant moon. Big and round. I wish I could enjoy it, but I can't. The clouds tried to brush it away, but that moon wouldn't let anyone push it around. It popped right out. And that's when I saw the man so clear under my bed."

Peg Harvey used visual words. She drew vivid, poetic pictures from the sky. I explored, matching her preferred sense. "Mrs. Harvey, when you see this man under your bed so clearly, what does he look like?"

"He has black hair, sticking straight up, like a broom turned upside down. He has bushy, black eyebrows bristling up and down when he looks at me." Peg stopped a moment to shudder. "He even has long, thin, black hairs coming through his nostrils, and little stubby whisker-like hairs coming out of his ears. He doesn't have a mustache, but he has a beard. The beard hairs are bushy, too, like his eyebrows. They stick straight out, from one ear to the other. He has the same thick stubby hairs on his chest." Peg stopped. Her picture image frightened her. She came close, whispering in my ear even though we were alone, "He has hair ALL OVER." Peg's teeth began to chatter. I could barely hear her frightened whisper, "He is naked, and *his thing is this big!*" Peg moved her two forefingers 5 inches apart, to indicate the length of his penis, shaking her head at its enormity.

I Centered, breathing deeply and slowly to silence chuckles that threatened to pop out of my mouth. Peg

Harvey would turn away from me if I laughed. She was deadly serious. She would spot a phony who found her funny. I would lose her trust.

Peg took my silence for disbelief. "Believe me, I am not exaggerating. If anything, I'm under-exaggerating."

I could not trust my voice to match her feelings, so I kept quiet. I needed to find empathy for her—fast! I remembered when I was 6 years old, playing "doctor" with Tommy, my blond, curly-haired friend who lived across the street. We were very serious, playing a game we invented that we called "Who's got what and where?" With toy stethoscopes snatched from our black, shiny, doctor kits, we examined each other. We had to remove our clothes in order to complete the examination. We ignored Dad's heavy footsteps. He opened the door to my bedroom: "MIMI! WHAT ARE YOU DOING?" He bellowed. He roared. His voice shook the chandelier. I trembled. What did I do wrong? "DON'T YOU EVER DO THIS AGAIN. TOMMY, GET OUT OF THIS HOUSE AND NEVER COME BACK! SHAME ON YOU. I'M TELLING YOUR PARENTS!" My old-fashioned father, who never used the word sex, smacked me hard across the face. My lip started to bleed. I was very ashamed. I wished to disappear from this earth. In high school, when my friends were experimenting in the back seats of cars, I sat prim and proper, my blouse buttoned securely. It took me years to untangle the fear-shame-guilt-sex knot tied together and locked up inside. With a spurt of empathy, I continued exploring to help Peg Harvey get rid of her sexual hang-up. "Mrs. Harvey, what do you do when it gets that big?"

"Nothing. I freeze and hope it goes down before something terrible happens." Peg's answer was matter-of-fact.

Without thinking, I asked, "Did something terrible happen to you that frightened you like this before?"

She snapped at me, "This has never happened to me before. You think I'm crazy. I am not in the habit of seeing naked men. Anybody would be afraid if all of a sudden they saw a man with that thing poking up."

I had made a mistake. I had tried to analyze her, to search her past to figure out why she was afraid of men. I wanted her to face her fear of sex, emotionally and intellectually. I was trained to offer people insight. I had to learn, again and again, that very old people can't use that part of my training. I had to abandon the goal of helping the very old victim find insight. I returned to the tried and true Validation technique of rephrasing. "Is his thing that big?" I asked her with respect. She nodded, her eyes widening. Her two forefingers moved apart another inch. I reflected her movement with my words. "Does he get even bigger?"

She answered eagerly, "That's when he pokes at me through the mattress, and you know what he wants." I nodded. We looked at each other, sharing common feelings. The moment ended. Peg got up briskly, her voice bright, her shoulders lifted, "Well, let's go back to the craft room. We've talked enough. I'll show you the cap I'm knitting for my grandchild. My children live in Vienna, you know. They work for the State Department." Peg changed the subject herself, relieved. She and I met twice a week, and each time we met I validated her. After several meetings, she stopped talking about the naked man with her friends, saving him for her talks with me and with the craft teacher. Peg knew that we would never ridicule her or withdraw from her. She knew that we believed her feelings. She trusted us. We were the parent-people who listened, who understood.

Her fears lessened. We charted the change in her behavior. Despite two full moons over the next 8 weeks, Peg

Harvey saw no man. And we never asked, "Mrs. Harvey, how is that man under your bed?" We talked about other things for 5–10 minutes each day, knowing that it was important to continue our relationship. One day, Peg confided to me. "Naomi, do you remember that man with the fuzzy black hair I told you about?" I nodded thoughtfully, careful not to smile. I had passed the test. She went on. "Well, he doesn't come anymore. Last night, there was a full moon, and he didn't come!"

"That's wonderful!" I said, joyfully. Peg peered at me through the top of her trifocals, changing her voice to a whisper. "Do you want to know what happened?"

I held my breath. "Yes!"

"Well," Peg said, settling herself in her chair, and leaning forward with relish. "Do you ever watch Channel 5 on TV?" I nodded, itching to find out the connection. But Peg was a story-teller. I had to wait for the end. "Do you ever watch the Lysol ad?" Peg didn't wait for me to answer. "Well, they advertise this super bottle of Lysol. It's special. You can't buy it at the supermarket. You have to call Channel 5. Do you know it cost me $23.99? And that does not include the shipping and handling, which cost an extra $3.95, but it was worth it." Peg smiled, changing her position in the chair, pausing. Satisfied that I was waiting with bated breath, she ended in triumph, "I sprayed that whole bottle under my bed, and that man hated the smell. He doesn't come anymore!" Peg was saving face. She had removed the man— but not forever. Peg lacked insight.

Later that year, she suffered a setback. Her daughter in Vienna had promised to visit her on Christmas. Peg had been counting on seeing her grandchildren before she died. She marked off each day on her calendar—only 5 days left. The day before Christmas, her daughter called to say the trip was off. The family had been transferred to Tunisia.

On Christmas day Peg saw one man after another under her bed. The loss of her daughter in present time had triggered the memory of an earlier loss, perhaps the loss of her sexuality. We had to validate her all over again. But we did not have to go back to the beginning. We had built trust. One week later, knowing that Peg felt safe with me, I used Validation Technique 5: imagining the opposite. This very effective technique works best after I have built trust.

"Mrs. Harvey, is there ever a time when there is a full moon and *no man under your bed?*"

Peg stopped rocking. "I never considered that possibility. You know, come to think of it, remember when you forgot your papers Tuesday night? It was about 10:00 P.M., and you saw that my door was open. Did you know that there was a full moon that night?" I shook my head. She continued. "Well, there was, a big orange one, full of holes. You stayed with me for about 10 minutes. Do you know that the whole time you were with me there was no man under my bed!"

I gasped. She nodded, sharing my wonder. "But," (and now came the punch line) "as soon as you left, he came back!"

I rephrased her words. "You mean, when I was with you, there was no man. But when you were alone, he came back?"

Peg stared at me. The clock ticked away the silence. "Do you think I'm lonely?" She had made a connection. Peg Harvey had tied her feelings to her needs. She had figured out a reason for the man under her bed—loneliness. But Peg would never gain insight into the underlying reasons behind her fears. Imagining the opposite was helping her think things through without threatening her. Asking Peg to imagine the opposite strengthened our relationship. If I had tried to get Peg to imagine the opposite when we first met, she would have answered, "The man always comes whenever there is a full moon. It doesn't matter who is with me." Without trust, Peg would not have been able to admit to me that she was lonely. I had to wait 3 months to build enough trust so that Peg would feel free to imagine the opposite.

Together, Peg and I faced her loneliness. We began to reminisce. Peg fluffed a few strands of her curly, pure white hair over one ear, like a schoolgirl. "You know, Naomi, I wasn't always lonely. I never had many friends in high school, just one, but that was enough. My husband was my only boyfriend. We met when he was 21 and I was 17. He came to me right out of the Army, tall, tanned, so handsome. He had lips that curved up when he smiled. Just before he died, he held my head in his hands and looked up at me from his hospital bed. So often, I see his eyes, clear and light brown, covering me, like a blanket, warm and safe. There was no room for anything else, just his soft, brown eyes." Peg ended with a deep sigh, full of longing, her eyes far away in romantic memory.

She was humming a catchy folk tune. "We sang together. Peter was on key and I was off key, but he didn't care. He loved me. We walked home from the movies, running up the hill to our new house . . ." Peg's voice broke. She shoved her memory away and stared at me, bleak and empty. Knowing that Peg could not handle too much intimacy, I never touched her cheek, but gently touched her arm with empathy.

Peg had been strong enough to survive her terrible loss at age 63. Perhaps she could recover enough strength to survive loneliness at age 82. I wanted to help her remember her earlier way of coping. It was too late to add new coping skills, but I could stir up some old ones. "What did you do to go on living when your husband died, Mrs. Harvey?"

"I couldn't live alone, Naomi. That's when I began seeing that horrible man under my bed. The one—you know—" Peg changed to her man-under-the-bed whisper. I nodded. Peg went on. "My best girlfriend from high school lost her husband about the same time, so she moved in with me. We cried together. We remembered kindergarten, and how we sent valentines to each other, how she met her husband, Tim. He was wearing a kilt at a party, and Patsy fell in love. We walked during the day and talked through the night, and that's how I got over my husband."

Peg Harvey looked at me with a new awareness. Her eyes did the asking, and I answered. "I would love to spend time talking with you during the day, Peg, but I'm only here 3 days a week. Do you think you could find a friend here who would enjoy looking at your photo album with Peter's pictures?"

She nodded. "You know Sophie Hale, the pudgy one with the rosy cheeks who always pokes her needle at you when she knits? She's really a nice person when she puts her needles down and you get to know her. Her husband died at about the same age as Peter. She misses him. She carries his picture under her dress, right near her heart."

Peg and Sophie stayed friends until Sophie died 3 years later. Peg died peacefully, 1 week after Sophie, without ever seeing the man under her bed.

STEWART, THE COMPLAINER: "YOU'RE KILLING ME HERE!"

Stewart Charkoff, age 81, was deaf in one ear. On even days, he wore his hearing aid. On odd days, he tuned everyone out. He had become "sick and tired of living with these old people in this old folks home with nothing to do." Arthritis gripped his knees, and he could no longer walk. He refused to be "hauled around on those iron thingamajigs," his name for wheelchairs. He resented being "mauled by those prissy nincompoops" who came to wheel him from place to place. Painfully, Stewart pulled himself up, each bone in his body creaking. Painfully, he reached for his walker, which somehow always escaped his grasp. He never cried for help. Moving arthritic fingers with the skill of a juggler, he attached the top of his cane to the foot of the walker. To go to the bathroom, he pulled himself up and pushed himself off.

"Mr. Charkoff, please, you shouldn't go to the toilet alone. You've been in the bathroom for 2 hours. Let me help you back to bed. It's 3 o'clock in the morning." The nursing assistant was worried. Stewart Charkoff had fallen from the toilet four times in the last 2 weeks. He poked the nursing assistant away with his rubber-tipped cane. "Get outta here, you asshole. She put poison in my tea, and I have to flush it out. I don't care if it takes 10 hours. I am not going to die in this hell hole. Now get away and let me be. I have to take care of my business." Stewart slammed the door to the bathroom. The nursing assistant sighed and complained to the head nurse.

The next morning, in the dining room, Stewart roared, "This tea is too hot!" The well-meaning waitress put ice in his tea. "What's this?" Stewart glared at her. "What did you put in my tea?"

"Ice—that's ice," the waitress explained, walking away to serve someone else.

Stewart caught her elbow with his cane. "Oh! No! You're not getting away with putting lice in my tea."

Exasperated, the waitress shook herself free. "I said 'ICE, not 'LICE,'" she shouted. "If you grab me like that, I'll report you for abuse."

Stewart was adamant and shouted, "Quit yelling at me. I heard what you said. I'm not deaf. You better take away those lice or I'll report you."

Everyone in the nursing home wanted to get rid of Stewart Charkoff. They called him "the menace." They were relieved when he was whizzed to the hospital in an ambulance. He had finally broken his hip reaching for his walker trying to get off the toilet. "Maybe he'll never come back," some of the aides whispered, giggling. They had been hurt too much too often. They had lost compassion for this angry victim.

In the hospital, Stewart Charkoff got worse. Totally dependent on the hospital staff, he became demanding. The nurses complained. "Your hand is never off the call button. We can't be running in here all day. We have other people who are really sick who need us. If you want service, get a private duty nurse."

Stewart turned to the telephone. He called the newspapers. "They're poisoning me in this hospital," he cried. "The public ought to know what they're paying for. I've put in Social Security for 63 years. I've paid for my rights to get a decent meal and decent service. You know what this lousy hospital room costs? The meals stink, and they poison my food. I haven't had a decent bowel movement since I got here." The hospital social worker called me to help. Mr. Charkoff had no children and had never married. Nobody was surprised. Who could live with him?

Unlike the other patients' doors, the door to Mr. Charkoff's room was closed. The nurses wanted to shut him out. His insistent call button kept ringing. Often, they ignored him. "Physically, he's fine," they told me. "Mentally, is another story. We are an acute care facility, not a psychiatric institution."

I entered with caution. Stewart Charkoff looked up with suspicion, dropping the call button. Pushing himself up, he leaned on his elbow to stare at me. "Well, you finally got up off your fat ass to see if I was dying? You're trying hard, but I'm not dead yet! One more meal like the last one, and you'll have the body. You want to use my parts while they're still warm? If you keep poisoning me, I won't be good to anybody, dead or alive!" He waited, expecting me to argue. Instead, I sat down near his good ear, took a deep breath to Center and rephrased his own words.

"Mr. Charkoff, you say they are poisoning your food?" I asked.

"Are you deaf, lady? Can't you understand plain English?" Stewart Charkoff peered at me disgustedly, amazed at my stupidity. I swallowed, Centered, and acknowledged my hurt. My father had used the same words, often, when I was 16. I searched for Stewart's preferred sense. Perhaps his taste buds were damaged, a big loss for a man who loves to eat.

"Mr. Charkoff, does everything taste awful here? Is it worse here than in the nursing home?"

"The food over there is just as bad. I told the newspaper what goes on." His anger was subsiding as he talked it out.

I tried using Validation Technique 4: asking the person to think about the worst case. "When is the food the worst? Breakfast, lunch, or dinner?"

"That's a good question, lady. That cook is a genius with chemicals, because each meal tastes worse than the other. I've had lousy cooking in my life, but this place tops 'em all."

Stewart Charkoff was beginning to reminisce. Moving gently, I explored his past. "Was your mother a good cook, Mr. Charkoff ? Did she make goulash with paprika?" I had a Hungarian husband who loved this dish, so I pulled it out for Stewart Charkoff.

"You must be Hungarian!" he said, chuckling to himself.

"You can spot a Hungarian. It's my husband, not me. Were you born in Hungary, Mr. Charkoff?"

Surprised, he nodded vigorously, "Yeah! If anyone knows Hungarians, it's me."

I continued questioning him gently, carefully avoiding the word, "why." I did not want to threaten this suspicious old man. My voice held respect for Stewart's wisdom, born from a lifetime of experiences. I always used his last name, aware that his generation used first names with children and peers only.

"Mr. Charkoff, were you a little boy when you came to Cleveland?"

"My father and mother brought me here when I was 10. They couldn't speak a word of English, but I learned fast. I'm what you call a 'landscape artist.'"

He raised his eyebrows in appreciation of his craft.

I raised mine, matching his movement, genuinely reflecting his feeling of accomplishment. My tone mirrored his pride.

"Mr. Charkoff, who taught you how to become a landscape artist?"

"My father. And his father before him. My people were not Gypsies. We owned land in Hungary. We knew how to work! You should have heard my father yell at us. At 5 o'clock sharp, every morning, when the cock crowed, he got us up." Stewart Charkoff raised himself, frustrated by his broken hip.

"It's a hard pill to swallow, to stay in bed when you've worked all your life. That makes you angry, doesn't it?" I said, trying to acknowledge his feelings. "That's the way it is," he said coldly. His voice became flat, bitter, and resigned, and he tuned me out. Like other Maloriented people, Stewart Charkoff did not want to be faced with his feelings. He denied feelings. He did not want to change his behavior. Confronting him with the consequences of his acting-out would destroy our budding relationship. If I would ask him, now, to stop swearing at the doctors and nurses, he would tell me where I could go and what I could do with myself when I got there. I was stuck. Ending our first interview badly could prevent the establishment of trust. Again, I tried Validation Technique 12: using the preferred sense. Perhaps hearing, not taste, was Stewart Charkoff's preferred sense. In addition to denying his feelings, Stewart had also denied his hearing loss. He had asked me if I was deaf. He had used hearing words to describe his father. I tried to speak his language. I used hearing words. "Mr. Charkoff, did you always listen to your father when he spoke to you?"

Stewart's voice lifted as he remembered. "Damn right, I did. I knew what he'd do if I didn't—out came the razor strap. But he was a good man. He wanted to do right by us. To this day, I can hear him. He gave everyone holy hell when they didn't listen to him!" Stewart Charkoff's appreciative chuckles mounted to a rip-roaring clap of laughter. He was remembering something specific.

"What do you hear him say, Mr. Charkoff?"

"He told that son-of-a-bitch teacher to keep her goddamn hands off my hair." He slapped his thigh with pleasure.

"What happened?" I wanted him to keep talking.

Stewart Charkoff gave me a sharp look, checking to see if I was really interested. I was. He went on reminiscing.

"Once a week, she checked our hair. She was looking for lice. She found some on me. She told all the kids: 'Stewart has lice. Don't go near Stewart because lice crawl from one head to another.'" Suddenly, his voice was quiet. "You know, no kid went near me for months. I was isolated. In solitary confinement. That teacher finally called on us and told my parents I had lice. My mother scrubbed my hair with kerosene. But my father told the teacher what she could do with her lice."

There had been a good reason behind Stewart Charkoff's hearing the word *lice* instead of *ice* in the dining room. Loss of his hearing had isolated him, just like the lice in his hair had when he was in the eighth grade. The feeling of being in solitary confinement was the same. His mounting losses in present time had sparked the memory of the lice. Again, similar feelings attract. They float through time and attach. Stewart Charkoff, alone and useless, overwhelmed by the loss of everything that mattered to him, had become a victim.

In the next 5 days, Mr. Charkoff and I talked. We spent 10 quality minutes each day. Stewart's hip mended. According to the nurses' reports, he had calmed down, and tranquilizing medications were no longer indicated. In the nursing home, we kept up our talks. To help him get rid of so much anger, I often used Validation Technique 4: using polarity.

"Mr. Charkoff, what is the worst thing about living here?"

His answer was swift. "Having nothing to do. Sitting in this chair like a goddamn idiot."

Stewart began to look for something to do. He wanted to work and was sad that he could not. To help him accept this loss, I used Validation Technique 5: imagining the opposite, and Validation Technique 6: reminiscing.

"Was there ever a time in your life when you couldn't work?" I asked.

Stewart thought carefully. "My father died during the Depression. I couldn't find a job." "What did you do?" I asked, gently.

"I went to the Government. They sent me with a gang to dig the foundation for a new hospital in Pennsylvania. I'm a landscape artist, not a ditch digger. My father would have tanned me good with his strap if he had seen me with a rusty shovel." His voice was bitter.

I persisted, wanting him to compromise, to accept his losses with less rancor, to find dignity in his life despite his sores.

"Did you quit, Mr. Charkoff?"

"Hell no! I couldn't quit. I would have starved."

"Don't quit, now, Mr. Charkoff. Don't starve yourself." I stared at him, knowing that he would understand my meaning.

"I'm not starving myself, it's that goddamned cook in the kitchen. I can't eat her slop."

Rephrasing, I moved toward finding a creative solution. "You can't eat her slop, and you don't want to be here, but you are here. Do you think you and I could go to the head of this place and ask for some work for you like you did during the Depression?"

It took 6 more weeks. I introduced Stewart Charkoff to the gardener, who was not Hungarian, but who, like Stewart, loved the land. The gardener became a member of my Validation team. In the spring, he helped Stewart steer his walker to a little plot of land nearby. From my office, I could hear him boss the gardener. "Hey, Charley, that's too much topsoil. Petunias can't stand that much."

Chapter 11

Communicating with
People Who Are
Time Confused

DAVID, THE TOUCHER: "I AM NOT DR. WILLARD. HE'S ON AN EXTENDED HOLIDAY!"

"I'm going to report him for sexual abuse!" Clara, the nursing assistant, tossed her head and pursed her lips. "He's a dirty old man, pure and simple."

"He's not so pure, and it's not that simple," Linda, her friend, giggled in answer, cupping her hand over her mouth to hide her laughter from the Director of Nursing (DON). Linda ran toward her patient who was sitting on the toilet, hollering, "Help!" The DON, hand on hips, locked eyes with Clara, who immediately blushed and looked down.

"Well?" asked the DON, in her clipped voice.

Clara sucked in her breath, squared her shoulders, looked the DON in the eyes, and said, defiantly, "I'm reporting Dr. Willard. He's grabbed my breasts for the last time. He's fast, I'll say that for him. They must have taught him in medical school just where to pinch. That is abuse. I could take him to court."

Clara went back to work in a huff, and the DON walked down to my office. Frowning, she sat on the edge of her chair. Together we reviewed Dr. Willard's history.

December 5, 1989: Dr. and Mrs. David Willard admitted to the nursing home. Mrs. Willard was oriented to time and place. Dr. Willard was diagnosed with Alzheimer's disease. They were placed in separate buildings. Mrs. Willard indicated that she did not want to be near her husband and was not interested in visiting him. She would not elaborate.

I looked up at Miss Jenkins, who had been the DON on the Alzheimer's floor for 10 years and who knew the residents and their families. I wondered about Dr. Willard's other family relationships. "Does their daughter visit?" I asked.

Miss Jenkins arched her eyebrows, punctuating each word with aplomb. "The daughter is Mrs. Elizabeth Whiting. Naomi, if you don't know the daughter, you've missed a treat. I've never been bossed around more by anyone in my life. *The* Whitings. Very well-to-do—real estate. Mrs. Whiting comes every day to see her mother and to tell me what to do for her father. But she never even says a word of hello to Dr. Willard, poor man. Naomi, you've got to do something. Dr. Willard is shaking up that young nursing assistant, Clara. I'm concerned that she's blowing this up all out of proportion, and it's beginning to affect her work." Miss Jenkins patted me on the shoulder for good luck and bustled back to work.

Dr. Willard's voice boomed at me from inside his room. "Come in, honey! I've got something you'll like. I can stick it right in." His bare feet dangling on the floor, he was sitting on the edge of his bed, searching for something in his night table drawer. I had knocked loudly, knowing that he was deaf in his right ear and that he refused to wear a hearing aid. David Willard winked at me as I approached him. Time Confused, he did not know that he had never met me before. In an instant, he had incorporated me into his world.

"Don't worry, honey, I'll find it later. I've got plenty of time." He smoothed the space next to him, patting it, jerking his head at me, indicating that I should sit down.

I smiled, sat down where he indicated, and shook his hand to introduce myself. "I'm Naomi Feil."

"Sweetie, I can run a mile, too. We'll do it together," he snickered, rubbing my breast insistently with his elbow.

Stifling a smile, I repeated, "My name is Feil." I stood up slowly, so as not to surprise him. My voice was gentle. "Dr. Willard, do you mind if I pull up a chair?" I sat facing him.

He chuckled, undaunted by my move. "Smile awhile with honey Feil." His high-pitched, crackly voice reverberated. He looked like a leering, nonmenacing crow. His thin arms flapped at the elbows. He cocked his head from side to side, sharply examining me from top to toe. David Willard was 93 years old, but his thick white hair was streaked with black clumps. His bulbous nose, nostrils flaring, dominated his thin, bony face. He hunched his shoulders, erasing his neck, squinting at me with beady, twinkly brown eyes, daring me to take him seriously.

"Dr. Willard, were you looking for something important when I came in?" I began, my voice sober, respectful.

He ignored my question, reached close, and pinched my cheek with one hand while rubbing my neck with the other. "How do you like them bananas, huh, honey bunch?" he cackled.

Gently, I removed his hands and laid them on his knees. I bent down to meet his brown eyes. Dr. Willard weighed 103 pounds, and his eyes held humor, not malice. I began again. "Dr. Willard, do you know that you are making me feel uncomfortable?" My voice was soft. Did Dr. Willard know what he was doing, or was there so much brain damage that he had lost his self-awareness?

"Am I making you feel uncomfortable, honey bunch?" Although partially deaf, Dr. Willard mimicked my voice-tone with perfect pitch. Then, in his own cackly voice, he confided, leaning close, breathing hard into my ear. "I am not Dr. Willard. David Willard is in his office, practicing medicine."

I did a doubletake and scratched the back of my neck to regain composure. Perplexed, my voice managed a concerned "Oh?" without breaking. In a respectful, matter-of-fact voice, I asked, "Well, who are you?" feeling a little like Alice in Wonderland.

He ignored my question, cocked his head, pointed to his scrotum, and cackled, "I've got a lovely bunch of coconuts just for you!"

I nodded, acknowledging his offer. Suddenly, he became serious, bent his head close to mine, and whispered, "David Willard is a very busy man. His nurse has his operating schedule. You must make an appointment with her. But I'm afraid you're too late. He's gone." Dr. Willard looked away, shutting me out to rummage in his drawer.

Suddenly, I felt sad, weighed down, depressed. Tentatively, I asked, "Do you think he'll ever come back?"

David Willard remained silent. His brain was no longer informing him of his body's whereabouts. He no longer knew where he was or who he was. He had put himself outside himself, picturing the well-known surgeon, wearing his laboratory coat in his office, practicing medicine. His controls gone, his self-awareness gone, Dr. Willard was releasing his sexual urge by pinching women without restraint.

"Do you want to see your wife?" I asked. Dr. Willard stopped rummaging in the drawer. I looked straight into his eyes. He averted his eyes, slid off the edge of his bed, and pulled the drawer from the nightstand, dumping the contents on the floor. He peered under the bed, into a corner, then opened the closet—his movements quick, urgent, frantic. He ignored me. I said goodbye softly and left.

Martha Willard, 84, sat straight up in her chair. Her sharp, blue eyes were cold. Her red-lacquered fingernails drummed lightly on the nightstand. Her newly styled hair was fashioned in the latest mode, tinted white-blue in an exquisite bun. Aristocratic portraits of Martha Willard's family hung decoratively on the walls; her father, mother, sisters, brothers, and daughter, in silver frames, smiled graciously. Her husband was missing. "You have a very handsome family, Mrs. Willard," I opened the conversation. "Your daughter is beautiful. She looks like you—the same even features."

"You don't have to compliment me. I know why you're here. My husband is doing awful things. I have no control over him. He is not my responsibility. That man never paid any attention to me. Now, it's too late."

I was taken aback by her frankness. Sucking in my breath, I explored. "What do you mean, 'it's too late,' Mrs. Willard?"

Her response was sharp and pointed. "I should have left him the first year we were married. In 65 years of marriage, he never showed a shred of emotion. Maybe it's all coming out now. He was a bland, cold man. He didn't want a wife, he just wanted to be married because a doctor is supposed to have a wife. He loved his work, not me. He wanted a child, not because he wanted to be a father, but because his mother wanted a grandchild. I've told you everything you need to know. I have no more to say." She looked at me intently, raising her eyebrows. She dismissed me by turning to her book. I left.

Elizabeth Whiting was beautiful, but her luminous hazel eyes reflected embarrassment. Her hands fluttered. "Mrs. Feil," she said. "I don't want to hide anything from you. My mother is very happy at Sunshine Villa. She's made friends here. She wants nothing to do with my father. I don't want to rock the boat. I arrange everything for him. Ask Miss Jenkins. I see to it that his suits are always pressed, he sees the barber every day. Just recently he got a costly new pair of dentures."

"Do you see him often?" I asked her, gently.

She averted her eyes, quickly inspecting her fingernails. Finally, she looked up. Her voice quivered a little. "I can't look him in the eye. My father was never around for me or my mother. He was a famous surgeon, but when I almost died of pneumonia, he was too busy taking care of his patients to see me. When Mother got appendicitis, she almost died. Father saw her in the hospital only *after* the operation. Even his doctor friends couldn't understand why he didn't rush away from patients who were strangers to take care of his own wife.

"Now, he's a dirty old man. That is the height of irony. He never showed Mother any kind of love. I never even saw them kiss. And I really don't think he ever fooled around with other women. He was always at the hospital, working. It's weird that at age 92, he's letting it all out, making a fool of himself, embarrassing everyone. I feel sorry for the nurses. He's taking it out on them."

"With us, he was an uptight, unfeeling human being. Mother stayed with him for my sake. I wish I had had the sense to help her leave him when she was still young enough to make a new life for herself. She was a wonderful mother. I love her very much. I know how deeply my father has hurt her. Now, she's beyond being hurt. She doesn't care what he does."

Elizabeth Whiting's voice broke for a moment. "He never came home for dinner unless it was a party for his doctor friends. We couldn't even make an appointment with him in his office. I don't think he wanted a family. He certainly didn't want us." Her voice turned cold. "I can't stand him. I can't look at him. I check up on him to make sure that his needs are met, for my sake, not for his. He is my father, and I owe him that."

I sighed. Neither mother nor daughter could help David Willard. My next move was to talk to Clara, the nursing assistant. Clara was cute, with short black hair and chubby, red cheeks. She was 18 years old and had just finished high school. For the past year, she had worked as a nursing assistant. Both her father and her mother worked in a local leather factory to support their seven children. Clara was the middle child. Her voice complained, not quite ringing true. "Naomi, you should have been there. You wouldn't believe how hard that little man can pinch. When they get old, some of them get mean. That man has strong fingers and sharp nails. He may be skinny, but when he gets going, watch out!"

I nodded, knowing what she meant. "Does he frighten you, Clara?" I asked quietly.

"Would you like to be pawed and pinched every time you get near someone? He has a long reach. I wish they would tie him up, or give him some medicine to calm him down. Just because he doesn't yell or wander out of the building doesn't mean that he shouldn't be restrained." Clara eyed me sidewise, checking my reaction, afraid that she might have gone too far. Her anger seemed to be out of proportion to David Willard's feeble attempts at seduction. I asked her in a quiet, matter-of-fact tone, "Clara, do you think that Dr. Willard knows what he's doing? Do you think he can control himself?"

"You better believe it!" Her voice was emphatic. "He knows exactly what he's doing. They all do. I can smell a dirty old man a mile away. I've known them since I was a little girl." Clara's voice held smug conviction.

"You have? How awful! What happened to you?" My reaction was spontaneous.

"Well, we had to pass this railroad track to get to school, and these drunks would chase us. Once, one of them caught up with me. I saw the look in his eyes."

"Clara, does Dr. Willard look like those men?"

Clara looked up, visualizing Dr. Willard. She frowned, concentrating. "No. Actually, he looks just like my Uncle Stanley. Dr. Willard has the same color hair, white with lots of black streaks, and the same hands and fingernails. I always notice their nails. Uncle Stanley had his nails polished, too."

"Did your Uncle Stanley disgust you, too?" I asked, quietly.

Clara looked at me quickly, her eyes full of surprise. Her mouth flew open in shock. She answered me slowly, each word loaded with awareness. "Yes. Uncle Stanley was a dirty old man, just like Dr. Willard." Clara spat out her words, her anger growing, unleashing. "My Uncle Stanley had that same slimy look—so does Dr. Willard. Whenever I bent down, Uncle Stanley would reach under my dress and feel around with his scratchy, lacquered nails. My mother didn't believe me when I told her, because Uncle Stanley was my father's oldest brother and loaned us the money for our house. I never had the nerve to tell my father. He would have called me a liar. I had to protect myself, all by myself. Naomi . . ." Clara began and then stopped talking. Her eyes clouded with sad memories and tears.

I sighed, remembering my own suppressed anger that suddenly found the light of day when a bitter 80-year-old resident reminded me of my father. I paid the price of self-awareness, too.

Clara was stung by feelings. She began to speak slowly, forming each word with sudden insights. "I didn't know it, but Dr. Willard brought out the anger I had to keep inside when Uncle Stanley pawed me. I felt so embarrassed, so awful, so mad. I guess it was not being able to do anything, knowing that no one would listen. Do you understand, Naomi?"

I nodded, my voice full of empathy. "Most of us who work with very old people experience what you're going through. The residents remind us of people in our past, and we don't even know it, consciously. Sometimes we act toward the old people the same way we wanted to act toward our parents, but couldn't. With you, it was your Uncle Stanley. You couldn't tell him to leave you alone, so now your anger is coming out at Dr. Willard. It's very important to become aware, so that we can change. We are all human and frail, but we struggle to become aware in order to change and grow."

We shared a silent moment, looking at each other with understanding. Clara spoke first. "I understand myself a lot better now. I think I'll get along better with my boyfriend after today. Naomi, I know that Dr. Willard has brain damage, and that he's lost his controls and can't help what he's doing. He's not like Uncle Stanley; he doesn't want to hurt me. I kind of feel sorry for Dr. Willard. His wife is so bossy, and his daughter is so snooty. Poor Dr. Willard! Always bossed around." Clara's words poured out in a rush, one thought tossing out another.

I gave Clara one more idea to take home. "Clara, sometimes families who can't communicate directly with their relatives dump their frustrations on staff. Mrs. Whiting seems snooty, but maybe she's afraid that she's not doing what a daughter should do, so she wants to make sure that the staff is doing everything possible. This way, families are reassured."

Clara got the point. "So that's why Mrs. Whiting keeps pushing me to buff Dr. Willard's nails and brush his hair and shine his shoes, even though I've told her a million times that he pinches me every time I bend down?" I didn't have to respond. Clara smiled, sprung lightly from her chair, and waved, reassuring me over her shoulder. "Don't worry, Naomi, I can handle 'Wiggly Willard' from now on."

"Clara, just one more question. Does Dr. Willard have a lady friend?"

Her hand over her mouth, she stiffled a giggle. "He sure does. He follows Melba Holiday like a panting puppy, carrying her purse like a newspaper. Where she goes, he goes. They're kinda cute. You know, she's the dumpy little old lady with the tremendous breasts. You always know when she turns a corner. Anything else? My boyfriend's waiting for me."

"No," I smiled at Clara. "Have fun!" She shot out of my office.

I included Melba Holiday in my Validation group, where residents sat close, held hands, danced, and swayed together. We sang love songs in the group and talked about needing love and affection. These wise disoriented old-old human beings helped each other solve the universal problem of loneliness. They met each other's need to unleash strong emotions. All through the day, the staff made sure that Melba Holiday sat next to David Willard. They held hands; she served him juice and cookies; they danced together and touched in a socially acceptable way. Within 6 weeks, David Willard was no longer pinching the staff as often. One week before he died, I visited him in his room. He was sitting in his usual position, on the edge of his bed, legs dangling on the floor, rummaging in his nightstand drawer. "Dr. Willard, can you not find what you are looking for?" I asked.

David Willard leaned over to stare at me, locking my eyes. He said simply with deep conviction, "David Willard is not here. The drawer is empty. I'll never find him."

David Willard's search for his identity came too late.

MARGARET, THE MOTHER: "I'M LIVING IN MY OWN HOME, THESE PEOPLE DON'T BELONG HERE!"

"Bethy, come home, honey!" wailed Margaret, loudly. She mumbled to herself softly, "Margaret, don't yell so loud! You'll disturb the neighbors." A moment later, she forgot herself once again. "Bethy was here just a minute ago. I hope nothing's happened to her. She turned that corner. Maybe she's playing with her friend. I have to get out of this chair, but there's a knot around my waist. I need a pair of sharp shears. Where did I put my sewing box? Wait! Thank God the knot's not too tight. I can slip right under. I better hurry, before it gets dark and Bethy loses her way. I should have asked Mother to take her. But Mother is always so busy, she doesn't have time for me or my children. *Bethy!* If I yell loud enough, maybe she'll hear me. She couldn't have gone far on her little legs. Bethy! Come home...right now! It's getting dark."

"SHADDUP!" "SHADDUP!" A chorus of voices chimed, one mimicking the other. "If that woman doesn't stop, I'll report her to headquarters," a 90-year-old former executive bellowed as he shuffled to the nursing station, pounding on the glass partition, demanding action.

Susan, the LPN on duty, was overwhelmed. "4 o'clock," she muttered, "and they all go crazy. Especially that Margaret. I wish they'd do something to calm her down. She's wearing herself out yelling." She turned to Hal, the 90-year-old man pounding on the window. "Hal, if you keep on pounding, you'll break the glass and cut yourself," she said.

Michael, the bearded, muscular orderly wiped the sweat off his chin with the back of his hand and moved toward the LPN to complain. "It's too hot on this floor. Why don't they turn up the air conditioning? By the way, I can't toilet three people at one time, and I am not bathing Hal. He weighs 210 pounds, and I can't lift him by myself. I don't want to get a hernia."

Susan nodded. "Can you just put Margaret back in her chair before you go. I'll toilet Hal. Poor Margaret! Her daughter took her doll away last week, and she's been acting nuttier by the minute. What's wrong with an 86-year-old woman holding a doll if it makes her happy?"

"She's not my mother, so the doll hasn't bothered me. But it bothers her daughter. I'll tell you one thing, I'm not getting myself sick on this job," said Michael. "Hey!

Margaret! Come back. You can't go out that door." Michael grabbed Margaret's sleeve as she tried to escape.

"Let her go, Michael, the door is locked," said Susan, sighing as she took Hal by the hand and escorted him to the toilet.

"Oh, yeah? Watch." Michael arched his eyebrows and folded his arms, releasing Margaret, who sashayed past. Unperturbed, she fiddled with the combination and slipped out the door. Michael followed with weary eyes, grumbling, "I knew it! She's figured out the combination. She's out!"

Margaret sped down the hallway, jabbering, "Bethy's probably looking for her little friend Tommy across the street." Margaret bumped into a wooden post. Her hands pressed the smooth, hard wood.

She used her mind's eye to picture her old neighborhood. "These trees were just seedlings when we moved here. Goodness, birch trees grow fast. Well, Margaret, you've lived in this neighborhood for 30 years. Everything grows older. Now, which way did Bethy go?" Margaret followed a railing that led to the elevator. She scooted inside the elevator just as the door closed. "They've changed the street all around. They put in this alley. No wonder Bethy gets lost all the time. You never know what they'll put in next. I better look on Chalfant—that's Tommy's street." Margaret slipped through the open elevator door toward the main exit as Michael grabbed her from behind. His hands tightened on Margaret's arms. Margaret shrieked. "LET ME GO! YOU TOOK MY BABY AWAY! LET ME GO! I HAVE TO FIND HER!"

"Now, Peggy, honey, I wouldn't take your baby. She's in her crib, safe and sound. Let's go back, and you can sing her a lullaby." Michael grasped Margaret's hand, pulling her gently as he spoke.

Margaret pulled free, dusting his fingerprints from her sleeve. She peered up at him, straightening as much as her hunchback would allow. Wagging a bony finger under his nose, Margaret hissed, "My name is not Peggy. It is Margaret. Mrs. Margaret Dowling. And my daughter is not in her crib. And I don't need you to tell me what to do—impertinent young man. Your mother should teach you how to behave with your elders." Her lips quivered. "No manners." Margaret clucked her tongue in disapproval.

"C'mon, grandma, don't give me any trouble. I should be home by now instead of wasting time with you." Michael had lost his limited patience.

Margaret admonished herself. "I am not listening to this young puppy. Margaret, you march yourself right out that door and find Bethy. The sun's down, and it's dark. She'll get lost. Get your hands off me!" she cried, as Michael grabbed her waist, pulled her into a wheelchair, strapped her down, and wheeled her swiftly into the elevator and back to her floor. He dumped her by the nursing station.

"I'm going home," he told the LPN. "She's all yours."

Margaret's breath came in small spurts. Blue veins splotched her neck. Furious, she shook her fist at the LPN. "I will have you arrested if you don't get me out of this chair immediately."

Susan turned her back on Margaret. By ignoring her, she hoped to stop Margaret's tirade. Perhaps this negative reinforcement might change Margaret's behavior.

"HELP! POLICE!" Margaret screamed at the top of her voice.

Susan telephoned the doctor, who prescribed Haldol, a tranquilizer. Two hours later, Susan called me, just as I was leaving for the day. "Naomi, come up to the floor right away. We had to quiet Margaret, so Dr. Finch prescribed a healthy dose of Haldol. Now Margaret won't wake up, and her daughter is furious."

"Mother, wake up. It's Molly." Molly Dunne gently pushed her mother's eyelids upward with stubby thumbs. Margaret's eyes would not focus. Her head slumped on her chest. She drooled. "This woman is not my mother. What did you do to her? She's a zombie!" Molly's voice cracked. She turned from her mother to look up at me, demanding an explanation.

"I wish I had an explanation," I said, my voice full of regret. At age 86, Margaret's system had reacted quickly to the medication. "Mrs. Dunne, can I meet you here at 4 o'clock tomorrow? Your mother always seems to panic around that time. Do you know why? Was 4 o'clock an important time in your mother's life?"

Mrs. Dunne had calmed down and was willing to talk. "Well," she said, "that's when we came home from school. Mother was very strict. None of us dared to be even 5 minutes late, except my sister, Beth. She was always late. Mom always worried. Poor Mom—look at her now. She looks dead."

The next day at 4 o'clock, Margaret was very much alive. "Mother," Molly pleaded, "Beth is a grown woman. She lives in Huntsville, Alabama. She has three children. You are a great-grandmother, for God's sake. You are 86 years old!"

Looking into space, Margaret ignored her daughter. She muttered over Molly's shoulder, "This woman acts as if she knows me. I won't pay her any attention. But I've seen her somewhere. She has a familiar face—nice eyes. Don had those same blue eyes and blond hair." The resemblance to her husband reminded Margaret of her husband, and her thoughts turned to him. "Oh, Donald, you died too young.

I knew you would die when you went to war. When I saw you in your uniform, you looked so handsome. I said to myself, 'Donald is going to die in this war. I will never see him again.' And you did. Beth has my eyes—small and squinty. Bethy is just like me, Donald. Molly is like you. That woman with the squeaky voice is talking to me. She squawks like a hen laying an egg. I better find Bethy before she catches cold. I think I feel a storm coming up. Get out of my way, Miss. I have to find my daughter."

"Mother," Molly groaned with hurt and frustration, "I am your daughter. It's me, Molly." Molly pointed to herself.

"Molly is my daughter. She's safe and sound. I have to find Bethy. She's out somewhere all alone in this storm. Get out of my way, please." Margaret poked Molly, sticking her elbows in her daughter's ribs.

"Mother, you're hurting me. Sit down. Beth is fine." Molly's voice was angry.

I moved close to Margaret, touching her gently on the back of her neck, adopting her voice-tone, picking up the rhythm of her breathing. "Are you worried about Bethy? What do you think will happen to her?"

"Oh, honey, she's all alone out there, in a terrible storm. Her father and I worry so much. She's just a little thing." Margaret moved toward the door with urgent, frantic energy.

I moved with her, gently touching her, mirroring her emotion. To put myself into her frame of mind, I thought of the time when my daughter ran into the street and almost got run over. "Where do you think she went? How far has she gone?" My worried voice matched Margaret's fear.

"Three long blocks . . . without a sweater in 30-degree weather," Margaret cried.

Margaret was visualizing her daughter, using her mind's eye, picturing little Bethy struggling in the snow. "What was she wearing, Mrs. Dowling?" I asked, using visual words to match what I perceived to be Margaret's preferred sense. Glasses never corrected Margaret's damaged optic nerve. Her outside world blurred. She moved inside, restoring people from the past like a painter repairing a faded portrait. Margaret moved in small, agitated steps. I fell in step with her rhythm. Her breath came in small spurts through her nose. I matched her breathing. Gently, I moved my finger tips on the back of her neck in a circular motion, a movement that often triggers memories of children. We moved toward the door together. I moved with Margaret, following her lead. I knew that the slightest pressure on her arm to turn her away from the door would spark a fight. She would resist, pushing me away, if I tried to lead. With my voice reflecting her fears and putting her feelings into words, we moved as one. "Do you think she fell in the snow? Did she have on her boots?"

"Of course she wore her boots!" Irritated at my stupid question, Margaret stopped to give me a scathing glance. "I would never let her go out without boots. What kind of a mother do you think I am?" Margaret's voice broke. She choked on her words. Grabbing my arm, she stopped dead in her tracks, her tone somber, low, and still. "It was a boy. I carried him for 9 months. Full term. He was fine inside for 9 months. He jumped in my stomach. I could feel him play inside me. I know he was healthy. He was ready to be born. They told me to hold in my baby until the doctor came. The doctor never came in time. My baby wanted to come out, but they held my legs together. My first baby boy. He came out half dead. He lived for 12 hours. When my roommate began to nurse her baby, my milk spilled. The pain digs a

hole in my chest, but I can't cry. My baby died. Full term."
Margaret looked through me, not seeing me at all. Cupping
her fingers, she gently placed her right arm in her left arm,
caressing it. She moved the right arm to her lips, kissing the
back of her hand, crooning. "My baby—here he is. He has
his father's beautiful straight nose—but my eyes. Lucky he
didn't get my long nose. He does look just like his dad. And
look at his dark hair. He has so much hair. The girls didn't
have all that hair. Shh. Don't cry, my baby boy. I'll sing you a
lullaby." Margaret held her hand-baby close, singing softly.
Her eyes filled with love, she sat to rock her infant.

I sat opposite her, bending close, gently placing my palm
over hers, mirroring her loving strokes. "You love your baby,
Mrs. Dowling," I whispered. "You worry so much about
your children. You want Bethy to be safe. You don't want
her to get hurt like your other baby. Is that why you worry
so much when it gets late and she's not home?"

Margaret Dowling stopped stroking her arm to look
me straight in the eyes. "Yes," she said. Sudden cognition
came over her. Fear and pain filled her body. She shuddered.
"I'm afraid Bethy will get hurt like my full-born baby." A
few tears came, then many, racking her body.

Molly took her mother in her arms, rocking her—
wordless. I caught Molly's eye. For the first time, she understood her mother's grief. Her eyes widened. "Oh, Mother,
that doll was your newborn baby. I took your baby away, for
the second time, last week. I didn't know you missed him
so much. You never cried when he died—your first boy.
I often wondered what happened. You never told us why
he died. Then Beth was born. I was always jealous because
you worried so much about her. You never worried about
me. But you always heard my tears. I love you, Mother. You
were a wonderful mother to us."

Margaret Dowling smiled at her daughter, tears forgotten. Her blue eyes lighting, Margaret took Molly's head in her hands, stroked a few stray strands of her daughter's hair, and whispered, "You are a wonderful daughter." Margaret turned to me. "And you are a nice girl. This is my daughter." Margaret patted my cheek. "And what's your name, honey?" Margaret had forgotten her daughter's name, but remembered her face. The 86-year-old woman had traveled 60 years in 60 seconds, moving through her lifetime. With my help, Molly learned to keep time with her mother. Margaret still looked for Bethy every day at 4 o'clock, but she had Molly to support her, and when she needed it, she had her doll.

HARRY, THE HITTER: "COME IN, YOU OLD BATTLE AX!"

"GODDAMN SONOFABITCH! GET OUTTA' MY ROOM!" Harry Tross narrowed his eyes, bared his teeth, and swung his cane at me. He leaned forward in his wheelchair, menacingly.

Instinctively, I Centered. To mirror his anger, I pictured myself stuck in the middle lane in heavy traffic, frustrated, helpless, trapped with nowhere to go. "Do you hate being stuck here, Mr. Tross?" I asked, matching his staccato, frustrated gestures with my fist.

Harold Tross split the air with a tremendous belch. "None of your goddamn business! Get out!" he bellowed. Harry had turned his former personality inside out. He had been a meek traveling salesman, selling stationery for 65 years. Reportedly "henpecked" by his wife, he had avoided his home and his responsibility as a father. His daughter felt sorry for him, but rarely visited. His wife could not understand his sudden violence. She lived alone in the community and wanted nothing to do with her formerly mild-mannered husband.

I wanted to build a trusting relationship with Harry Tross, to help him express his anger and relieve it so that he could make friends instead of isolating himself. I knew that without stimulation from the outside world, he would become one of the living dead in this nursing home. "You moved around all your life, Mr. Tross. In how many states did you sell stationery?" I asked.

Harry sneered at me, screwing up his lip, exposing his gums, a red valley among three yellow teeth. "You are the ugliest woman I have seen in a long time."

Hurt, I Centered again. My voice quivered. "Your territory included Ohio and Pennsylvania, didn't it?"

Harry Tross pursed his lips, narrowed his eyes, leaning forward. He crooked his finger, motioning me close. I took a chance, hoping that I could catch his cane if he should strike. I moved in 2 feet, bent down to meet his eyes, and moved my hands slowly toward the arms of his chair. Whack! Involuntary, tears blurred my vision. I jumped away. Outrage swept through my body. My hand stung, pulsing with throbs of pain. I breathed slowly, in and out, continuing to Center until the pain subsided. My hand would soon turn black and blue. (Life is colorful in a nursing home, I thought.) My sense of humor restored balance. I looked at Harry Tross. His eyes held torment.

"Goddamn Harry. Hari-kari. Harold Tross, shut up!" His deep voice rumbled, catching in his throat. He stopped suddenly, caught his breath, and seemed to shrink, folding himself into his chair. His head slumped on his chest, shoulders curved together, feet tucked tight, he shrank, a mean scrap of humanity in a wheelchair.

"Do you feel bad when you hurt people?" I asked, wanting to put his feelings into words.

No answer. Harry Tross had become a lifeless lump of flesh, almost invisible. He turned his chair toward the wall. Harry Tross dominated our staff meeting. We showed each other our "Harold Tross bruises." The male nurse pointed out, "He never hit me. I think he only hits women, because he hates his wife. And, I don't blame him. She is a bitch!" At age 82, weighing 110 pounds, Harold Tross's system would not tolerate high dosages of tranquilizing medications. My assignment: Talk to Mrs. Tross. Find out if she could help her husband.

Helen Tross had a mustache. She breathed hard, ruffling the fine hairs. She dyed her thinning hair orange to match her lipstick. "Mrs. Feil, I live 2 miles from here, and I don't drive a car. I had to take a cab here. That is quite an imposition. I am not a young woman, you know. I won't tell you how old I am because you won't believe it—nobody does. Ask me!" Her smug smile revealed well-matched dentures. I opened my mouth to ask, but was interrupted before I could speak.

"I am almost 80 years old. Isn't that something? My mother lived to be 98. She was some woman." Mrs. Tross paused to remember her mother.

I seized the moment. "Mrs. Tross, your husband is giving us a lot of concerns. He is becoming more and more violent. We know that he reacts poorly to tranquilizing drugs, so we don't want to medicate him. Can you help us?"

Mrs. Tross's eyes widened, incredulous. "My husband? Violent? That man was afraid of our cat. I put him in here because he couldn't find his way from the front lawn to the door of our house. He got lost putting out the garbage. He is so afraid of people he wouldn't answer the door. How he ever worked as a salesman is beyond me. Lucky my parents left me something. All he left me is a pile of headaches. You called me here to ask me to fix him up?" Helen Tross laughed cruelly, tossed back her head, and put on her coat. "And I thought you got me here because he left me some more money. Will you call me a cab?"

Mrs. Tross had failed to help us. We were on our own. We tried behavior modification. Whenever Harry hit out, became abusive, or used obscene language, we isolated him. When he refrained from verbal or physical abuse, we rewarded him with special attention and extra desserts. Our efforts were in vain. Harold Tross continued to strike out.

My heartbeat quickened when I knocked on his door the next week.

"Come in, you old battle ax!" he cried.

His raspy voice reached the pit of my stomach. A little voice inside me whispered, "This is not the right time. Tell him you'll come back later. You have to go to the bathroom." I smiled, recognizing the voice of fear. I breathed in and out. Letting my stiff, hunched shoulders relax, I felt my arms swing free. Now, I was ready to greet Harold Tross.

He taunted, his tone sarcastic. "Why don't you give up, lady? Can't get enough of me, huh, bitch?"

"Mr. Tross, I will not take any more of your swearing," I said calmly. My voice was even. I turned my back to walk out of his room. His shoe flew out the door, just missing my left ear. Over the next 2 weeks, we tried different types of behavior modification. Harry's aim improved.

One day, a young nurse met me on the unit floor. "Naomi," she said, "we won't need to tranquilize Harry Tross." She pointed to his room. "Look inside."

I gasped. Harry had squeezed his head through the narrow space that separated the back of his chair from the seat.

His arms dangled, lifeless. He had put himself in a stockade. He looked nowhere, with numb eyes. Over and over, he chanted solemnly, "Hari-kari. Hari-kari. Harry Tross, shut up." I bent down close to him and echoed his chant. He focused, seeing me for the first time. His eyes filled with shame. A moment passed—he began to sing. "Up in the air, junior Birdmen. Up in the air, upside down," his voice blasted. Imprisoned by his chair, his arms plunging up and down, he mimed the motion of an airplane, hollering: "We are the Army Air Corps." He slashed the floor, hitting it hard.

"Mr. Tross," I asked, "are you flying an airplane?" No longer aware of present time and place, his controls gone, Harold Tross was using his chair to replay his past.

"You're goddamn right, I can fly this plane. But I can't fly outside the plane. I'm dead, lady. I died last year... a thousand deaths," he answered swiftly, making poetic sense. "Hari-kari. It's the only way." He twisted his head, jerking his body violently back and forth, pulling his chair downward, wanting to hit the floor.

I bent down with him, filled with his grief. "Mr. Tross, do you want to commit hari-kari? Are you so ashamed?"

"Yes," he whispered.

I watched a tear find its way to his cheek. Gently, I wiped it. Harry closed his eyes and wept. In this moment, the seeds of trust were laid. Harry became the drummer in our Validation group rhythm band. Slashing the drum with his fist, riding his rage, he got rid of some of it. He was never easy to deal with, but he stopped throwing shoes. He and I talked often about his wife, his work, his regrets. We smiled a lot. I loved talking to Harry Tross. He made my work lighter. He gave me joy. And he outlived his wife.

VALIDATING AT HOME: KARL, THE FLASHER

Karl Madson adored his wife. She was the light of his life. They met when Karl was 25 and Hazel was 23. He was an accountant, and she was a bank teller. It was love at first sight. Karl was a virgin when he married Hazel. He had been tempted as a 19-year-old soldier on leave in Paris. With his army buddies, he ogled prostitutes in bordellos, but always "chickened out" at the last minute. Hazel had flirted. She had an affair at age 17 with a Navy officer whose ship was later torpedoed in World War II. Without Hazel, Karl would have floundered. She supported him, encouraged him, and dominated him. He rose to chief accountant. Hazel lovingly, but with a firm hand, raised their two children. When their girls married, the couple grew closer. Puttering with daily chores as years flew by, they had few friends and never traveled.

Each had his or her own routine. Karl played bridge on Tuesday nights; Hazel studied yoga. Neighbors smiled, poking each other, peering through curtains, a bit envious, watching 75-year-old Karl hold his wife's hand as they strolled home from church every Sunday. At age 85, Karl began to lose track of days. He wandered to the bank at 1:00 A.M. demanding his job back. The police brought him home, warning Hazel that he was disturbing the peace.

Hazel watched him night and day. At the supermarket, Hazel heard a gasp. She turned to find Karl unzipping his fly and pulling out his penis. Stunned, flushed, and fuming, Hazel dropped her groceries and dragged Karl into the street.

Contrite, unaware that he was acting inappropriately, Karl took Hazel's hand, tottered by her side, and was subdued and docile.

At her wit's end, Hazel scolded Karl, "Karl, aren't you ashamed of yourself. How can you behave like that? What am I going to do with you?" Karl blinked away a tear threatening to dribble down his cheek. "I love you, sweetheart. I don't want to hurt you." "You are hurting me. You are killing me. If this keeps up, I'll have to put you away." Hazel pounced, slapping Karl's hand, her eyes flaming.

The neurologist found "severe arthritis, increasing brain atrophy, a score of 19 on the Folstein Mini Mental Status Test." Karl was diagnosed as having an Alzheimer's-type dementia. The neurologist suggested nursing home placement.

Hazel's heart ached. At 3:00 A.M., while Karl wandered aimlessly from room to room, Hazel cornered him. "Karl, we can't go on this way. Either you behave or you'll have to live in a nursing home." Karl kissed her and promised to behave. But Karl couldn't behave. He had lost his social controls. He had lost self-awareness and cognition. He was not aware that he was losing sexual inhibitions. He had moved into the final life struggle: Resolution. In Time Confusion, his sexual feelings repressed for a lifetime surfaced. He had worshipped Hazel. She was a goddess. He had always controlled himself in bed. He had never abandoned his strict moral code; he couldn't give himself to her without restraint. In old age, unfulfilled desire demanded fulfillment. If Karl had released his sexual drives as a young man in France, he never would have acted out sexually as an old man in Kansas. He would have expressed his emotions throughout life. Sexual longing would not have built up, lurking inside for so many years, waiting to erupt. Hazel loved Karl quietly, without passion. Her love was enduring. Sex was acceptable but not fun with Karl. Only once, when they were first married, did she have an orgasm. At age 83, Hazel had grown accustomed to a meager sex life. She felt no pangs of desire. She never spoke of sex to her husband. She didn't miss it. Now, she resented his loss of control; furious, she wanted to whip him at times. But she knew that he would deteriorate away from her in a nursing home. Hazel decided to keep Karl at home.

Embarrassed, but desperate, Hazel confided to her minister. Her head bowed in shame, she could not look Pastor Johns in the eye. The minister's mother had also been diagnosed as having Alzheimer's-type dementia. He had researched the field and had just returned from a Validation workshop in Lansing, Kansas. He handed Hazel a copy of *The Validation Breakthrough*. Every Sunday, Hazel attended the family support group that Reverend Johns had created at the church. Here, family members learned to Center, to accept their loved ones "where they are" to stop judging.

One Sunday, Hazel gasped with a jolt of sudden insight. Karl's mother, severe and forbidding, had taught him to "respect" women; that meant not to touch them. Early learning stays. Karl felt guilty when his sexual urge surfaced. He learned to mentally slap his hand at age 8. "No wonder he is suddenly touching me all over. Poor man. He could never be himself. He's so full of love. Now, it's all pouring out." Hazel's compassion and caring grew. "How can I expect him to act the way he did when I first met him. The man is 85 years old. His brain is damaged. His normal, human urges are coming out, and he can't control them. He doesn't even know what he's doing. I can't expect him to behave. But I can help him. I can be with him, inside. Feel the way he feels. Show him that he's not alone."

Hazel learned the 15 verbal and nonverbal Validation techniques. When Karl zipped down his fly in the supermarket, Hazel moved close, helping him tuck himself back. Hazel used Validation Technique 13: Touch. *Where* one touches is important. Karl wanted sexual love. Facing him, she gently stroked the side of his neck, moving her middle finger from his earlobe to his chin. She validated his human need with words, close to his ear: "You want sex now, is that right Karl? You feel that urge?"

The gentle stroking motion soothed him. His voice cracked with love, "I love you, sweetheart. I never want to hurt you. Never."

Quietly, hand-in-hand, the two moved home together as one. Rephrasing, using Polarity and The Preferred Sense (i.e., feeling words), Hazel helped Karl vent his sexual needs with words. He rarely needed to act them out.

At home, Hazel faced Karl on the couch, touching him once more on the side of his neck, asking softly: "Is your heart beating fast now Karl. Do you feel warm?" (She used the Kinesthetic Sense.)

Karl smiled and stroked Hazel's breast gently.

"That feels good, honey." Hazel moved closer.

Karl suddenly lunged at Hazel, now on top of her, shouting, "So you're the French whore? You better be good, baby. I'll show you how."

Hazel's inner voice came through loud and clear. Automatically, she Centered, breathing slowly until the shock subsided. Her inner voice continued: "Rephrasing always works when I don't know what to say." Listening to Karl's voice tone and the rhythm of his speech, Hazel picked up her husband's intonation, "Did that whore know how? Did you show her?"

"Damn right, I did."

"What was the best thing you did, Karl? What made you the happiest? (Using Polarity.)

Karl's eyebrows twitched. His eyes lit like a torch, twinkling in glee. His lips puckered. He curled his tongue. He whispered, cupping his hands over his mouth, telling a shameful secret, "I French-kissed her." Then he roared, slapping Hazel soundly on the knee.

Karl started to sing with gusto, moving away from Hazel, swinging his arms like a baton. "Mademoiselle from Armetiere, parlez-vous. Mademoiselle from Armetiere, parlez-vous. The Mademoiselle from Armetiere, she hasn't been laid in 50 years. Inky dinky parlez-vous!"

Hazel joined Karl, and the two sang World War II songs into the night, falling asleep in each other's arms.

Chapter 12

Communicating with People Who Are Repetitive Movers

ISOBEL, THE POET: "I UNTANGLE THE NOODLES IN THE MIRRORS OF MY MIND"

She peeked into dresser drawers, wastebaskets, toilet bowls . . . anything that might hold something. Her oversize housedress swished as she walked, pockets loaded with odds and ends. Her pale blue-green eyes glowed with anticipation, peering, poking. I watched her chubby form, enfolded in fabric, disappear behind the drapes. "What are you looking for, Mrs. Blue?"

"Honey," she smiled, her dentures clicking, "I'm looking for yesterday. I have to untangle the noodles in the mirrors of my mind."

I blinked, struggling to grasp her poetry. I rephrased. "You're untangling the noodles of your mind? Have you found them?"

"If I found them, I wouldn't be looking, would I?" she whistled, patting me on the cheek. "Fay, you have the sweetest fiddlemaker, but you filled that forman with swadlefellows, and that's why you can't heddle him," she confided in a rueful cadence, sighing a sad sigh.

"Does that make you sad?" I asked. I had no idea what Isobel was trying to say, but wanted to continue talking.

"Dear," she confided, "you pull those strings too hard."

"Oh! Am I pulling your strings too hard? I'm sorry." I wondered if I asked her too many questions.

"Honey, we all play different tunnels. You can't fiddle all the time. That man will fleck your undertomes no matter how hard you pitzzle him," her voice, warning me, held fear. Isobel's eyes narrowed into green-flecked slits. She pursed her lips and split the air with her hand, whacking an invisible something. "Ouch! That hurts!" she yelped.

From across the day room, Isobel's equally disoriented roommate made circular motions with her forefinger, pointing to Isobel's head, screeching, "She's nutty as a fruitcake! She's crazy!"

"It's better to be crazy," Isobel tittered, slapping her thighs, "because then it doesn't matter what you do!" She tugged the drapes, convulsing with glee.

The nursing assistant wagged a finger at Isobel. "Leave those drapes alone! That's naughty."

"I'll tell my mother on you!" Isobel flashed back, flicking her wrist at the nursing assistant.

"Isobel, sweetie, you are 88 years old. Your mother would have to be at least 110. Honey, she couldn't be alive."

Isobel shrugged. "Well, I know that, and you know that, but my mother doesn't know that, and she won't like it one bit when I tweddle her! I just had a wonderful squackle with my mother and my aunt, and I didn't have the heart to hittle them. It'll hittle them too hard to know that they're dead. And ..." Isobel tossed her head, hands on hips, in a final gesture, "... a lot of old people live a lot longer than younger people. So waddle out! Today you say; tomorrow, you're dead!"

The nursing assistant threw up her hands. I scurried off to find a pencil to preserve Isobel's warning.

Crooking her finger, Isobel motioned to me to join her in her makeshift office behind the curtains. I slipped in by her side. "Fay, you'll get swaddled if you keep mixing with that one." Isobel pointed to Harry Tross, sitting in his wheelchair nearby, tearing pieces of tissue. Isobel shivered.

"How do you mean, 'swaddled,' Mrs. Blue?" I mirrored her ominous tone.

Isobel whacked the air with her hand, her fingers stiff. Her sudden forceful movement frightened her. She trembled, hiding her body behind the folds of the curtain.

"Are you seeing the man who swaddled you?" I put an arm around Isobel to ease her fear. She nodded, holding me close. "Did he smack you with his hand, like that?" I mirrored her hand motion, thwacking the air. Isobel's eyes widened. "With a switch and a paddle," she whispered in my ear.

"Oh!" Isobel's meaning dawned on me. She had combined the words "switch" and "paddle" to form the word "swaddle." Blending words and images, Isobel freely moved her tongue, teeth, and lips, letting similar sounds create new words.

"Was it your husband who paddled you?"

Isobel shook her head, tears surfacing. "He makes me cry. He wants me to fiddle all by myself. Fay, I can't." Isobel's voice broke. She tugged at my sleeve, imploring, "I want to fiddle, but I can't. Tell him that."

"He wanted you to fiddle, but you couldn't?" I repeated. I bent down, studying her eyes. All my energy was focused on Isobel. She hung her head.

"I can't play. I'm no good. He pulled my strings and broke it."

"Your father wanted you to play the fiddle? And you couldn't, so that broke it?" My voice caught. Gently, I touched Isobel's cheek with the palm of my hand, nurturing her.

"Mother tried to heddle him, but she couldn't. Fay, you can't do it. It's a florid invention." Isobel looked into my eyes, somber.

"A 'florid' invention?" I asked.

"*Fluid.* Your eyes are watery. Fays don't cry," said Isobel, patting my cheek.

"Is Fay your mother?" I asked. Isobel called all the female staff "Fay."

"No. Fay. Fay Wray. Fay is anyone who knows anything. Fay can fiddle like a falstra."

I remembered that Fay Wray was a silent movie star, a heroine who survived. Isobel moved away from the curtain toward Harry Tross. Her body swayed, graceful and fluid. She stretched her hands, palms upward, toward Mr. Tross. "Daddy, don't swaddle me. I'll fiddle for you," she begged.

"You will, will you?" Harry Tross boomed. "Well, fiddle away, whore."

I rushed to get the rhythm band instruments, and we found a fiddle for Isobel. In the weeks to come Isobel would sometimes hide her fiddle behind the curtain, but more often, in the Validation group, she played. I never found out what happened between Isobel and her father. In the Validation group, backed by the group members, Isobel was able to tell Harry to stop calling her names. Two weeks later, at her birthday party, she pulled me close to whisper, "I'm a Fay, too."

MARY, THE PACER: "I AM NOT A SHEEP!"

Swish. Black slacks flew past rows of wheelchairs. *Smack.* Tennis shoes thumped the tile floor. *Hss.* Sharp spurts of breath warned innocent passersby. Fists tight, elbows jutting out, Mary Thomas splattered anyone in her way. Back and forth, like a caged tiger, she paced. Eyes screwed tight, lips pursed, head down like a bull lowering his horns, she scared everyone. She never looked up. Her eyes hugged the floor even when she ate. Her thick rubbery lips wobbled, releasing high-pitched bleats: "Baa. Baa. Baa."

"PIPE DOWN, BITCH!" Harry Tross bellowed and drowned her sheep sounds.

"Get me outta' here!," wailed a 102-year-old woman.

"Tell her to shut up!" chimed another.

"She's crazy. Put her in the insane asylum," ordered a former policeman.

Heedless, Mary Thomas bleated past them all. She came close to kicking the others in her size 11 sneakers, but she never touched. Mary traveled alone. The other residents kept their distance. No matter how many times we bathed Mary Thomas, she smelled. A pungent, sweaty odor seeped from her clothes into the day room. She needed no other protection.

"Naomi," wailed Darlene, my 23-year-old second-year graduate student, "I can't work with Mary Thomas, and it's not the way she smells." Darlene caught my surreptitious blink. "I've gotten over that. I spray the air with 'Lilies of the Field' whenever I go up there." Darlene, a saucy redhead from Minnesota, wrinkled her freckled nose and grinned. "It's . . ." Struggling to pinpoint her thoughts, Darlene stopped talking, twisting her fingers. She looked up, thinking. Finally, she admitted, ruefully, "I just can't like her. I know that I have to stay objective, but how can I do social work with someone who turns me off?"

"That's a good question." I nodded in sympathy. "Nobody, not even a professional social worker, can like everybody."

Darlene grinned, relieved.

"What turns you off the most, Darlene?" I asked.

Darlene lifted her chin thoughtfully, visualizing Mary Thomas pacing back and forth in the day room. "I think it's that she never looks up. It's as if her eyes are stuck in the underworld. How can I reach her if she doesn't want to be reached. She's always looks down, ignoring me!"

"Darlene, are you picturing Mary Thomas now? Can you actually see her feet?"

Darlene looked surprised, "Why, yes. She has holes in her sneakers and wears at least a size 11."

"Darlene," I smiled, "you are probably mainly a visual person. You prefer your visual sense. Do you dream in color?"

Darlene nodded emphatically. "I watch a color movie that I picture for myself every night before I go to sleep."

"That's great!" I admired Darlene for her visual skills. "Most of us have a preferred sense. To picture something, most people look up and to the right. Before you answer a question, you almost always look up. Are you aware of

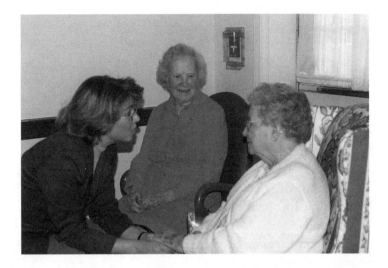

that?" Before answering, Darlene instinctively looked up. She smiled and nodded.

"Mary Thomas always looks down," I said. "That may mean she prefers her kinesthetic sense. Mary Thomas feels things. Her sense of touch is important. She thumps her feet, scraping the floor, hitting the road, probably enjoying the sensation. Mary is a person who feels before she sees or hears the outside world."

I wanted Darlene to step into Mary Thomas's shoes, so we reviewed her history. Diagnosed with Alzheimer's-type dementia at age 79, she had lived with her bachelor son for 5 years, ever since her husband had died. She had been admitted to the Alzheimer's floor the previous year after she threatened her son with a broom handle. He claimed that she was becoming violent and placed her in the nursing home.

Raised on a farm, the oldest of eight children, Mary never finished high school. Her only son, Malcolm, age 58, never understood his mother. She barely spoke to him. She did her duties—cooking, cleaning, laundry, sewing, shopping. Malcolm's father, a factory worker, expected his lunch pail ready on time, and Mary always did what she was told. Malcolm remembered one stormy Tuesday when his mother overslept. At 5:45 A.M., a sleepy Malcolm watched his father drag Mary out of her bed, shake an empty lunch pail in her face, and slap her. "She never forgot after that!" Malcolm assured us.

Darlene bristled, "Did your mother ever get to go on a vacation or leave the house to play bridge or spend time with friends?"

Malcolm shook his head. "She never had time," he answered simply.

"What made her threaten you with the broom?" asked Darlene. A feminist, she was gaining empathy for Mary Thomas.

"She hung a greasy shirt in my closet. She never washed out the stains on the collar. So all I did was give it back to her and say, 'Ma! you're supposed to get out all the stains. They tell you how on TV! She spit on my best shirt and started yelling, 'Baa! Baa!' She wouldn't stop. It drove me crazy. All I said was, 'Ma, quit it!' She shook the broom handle in my face. Then she took her shears and cut my best shirt into a hundred pieces. My best blue plaid shirt. There wasn't even a piece left over big enough for a handkerchief. Right after that she started her lousy pacing—night and day, back and forth, 'Baa. Baa.'" Malcolm wiped his brow with a dirty handkerchief.

Darlene went upstairs to Validate Mary Thomas. Mary was breathing hard, her bleats nasty blasts, hurtling anger. Darlene, the daughter of a "macho" father, still furious at her Dad, had no trouble empathizing with Mary. She mirrored

Mary's quick, fiery breaths. She paced with Mary, matching her sharp, staccato rhythms. Like two bulls, Darlene and Mary kept time.

"Now there's two of 'em," a resident roared.

"Put 'em both in the pen!" the former sergeant bellowed.

The LPN on the floor was part of our Validation team. She had experienced the effectiveness of mirroring. She tossed a bean bag at the resident and the former sergeant, giving Darlene room to mirror Mary's gait, to match her breathing, to duplicate the expression of her lower lip, and to reproduce the tonal quality of her bleating sounds.

Mary stopped short. She stared at Darlene. Darlene's eyes held compassion born of shared misery. Mary cried, "I'm not a sheep."

Using the palm of her hands, Darlene gently touched Mary's cheeks. "No, Mary," she said softly, "you're not a sheep, you don't have to do what everybody tells you. You are a person, Mary Thomas." Their eyes locked.

Slowly, Mary's lips formed the words "A person, Mary Thomas."

These were the first words that Mary had spoken in over a year. They were not her last. Mary Thomas continued pacing, but she rarely walked alone. A Validation team marched to the beat of her drum.

Chapter 13

Communicating with
Maloriented and
Time Confused
People Living in
the Community

THE APARTMENT HOUSE MANAGER, THE POLICEMAN, THE EMERGENCY MEDICAL SQUAD, AND THOMAS KONIG

"Mr. Konig? Are you in there? Mr. Konig?" The mild-mannered apartment manager's voice climbed a half note. Smelling trouble, he knocked with more force. In 9 months, he had had two dozen battles with the tenant in 14-B.

"GET THE HELL AWAY FROM MY DOOR, YOU PIPSQUEAK!" thundered a raspy voice from inside.

The apartment manager swallowed his fear. "Mr. Konig, you left the water on in the tub. We have to fix it. The ceiling is leaking in Mrs. Alderside's room. Please open the door."

"Screw Mrs. Aldertop! She could use a bath once in awhile, the way she stinks up the toilet," yelled back Mr. Konig.

"Mr. Konig," the manager persisted, sweating, "I'll have to call the police again. Remember last time, they broke your double locks, and your son had to pay?"

"It's about time that son-of-a-bitch paid me back for what I did for him. I'm not opening the door, for you or anybody else, so scram!" Thomas Konig jiggled the lock, shaking the door to assert his independence. To prove he meant what he said, he stripped and hopped into the overflowing bathtub. His 208 pounds whipped up a splendid deluge. A retired seaman, Thomas Konig loved water. "Oh, the ocean waves may roll, and the storm may blow, but we poor sailors go skipping to the top, and the landlubbers ..." Thomas Konig stopped singing to lean out of the tub and bang the floor with the handle of his scrub brush, yelling lustily, "Hear that, old lady watertop? The landlubbers lie down below. So shaddup!" He smiled, looking down at his neighbor below.

Thomas looked up into the eyes of the policeman. The officer, resigned after 10 years of trying to lay down the law to this ornery 80-year-old seaman, warned quietly, "You've disturbed the peace in this neighborhood long enough. You're going to the psycho ward." The police officer spoke to the two emergency medical technicians waiting to remove Thomas from his watery lair. "You can take him on the stretcher if he won't walk."

Thomas rose, water dripping from his naked body, his fists moving in circles like a boxer! "Get away from me. I'm only minding my own business. Why can't you people let me alone!" Not wanting to use restraints on the old man, the police officer tried logic. "Every night, at 2:00 A.M., we get complaints about you."

"Me?" Thomas gasped, astounded.

Patiently, the officer explained. "Last night at 2:12 A.M., you emptied three garbage cans on the sidewalk. You banged tin cans together and then you sang dirty Navy songs at the top of your voice. You howl worse than the alley cats."

"Nosy people. They should be sleeping, not listening to me. Why don't they mind their own business?" Thomas fumed, folding his arms in defiance. "I am not leaving this bathtub. And no one is going to make me!"

John Dawes, an emergency medical technician, was also a skilled Validation therapist. He used the Validation techniques for the Maloriented old person who holds on to worn out roles, who cannot face unpleasant emotions, who cannot tolerate old-age losses. John rephrased Mr. Konig's words, stressing the key word. "No one's going to make you do what you don't want to do, is that right, Mr. Konig?" John's voice held genuine respect.

"Damn right—on the button," Mr. Konig retorted, in grudging agreement.

"What do you want to do?" asked John.

"Finish my bath alone. Without you buggers nosying in my business!" he snapped.

Tom Konig stood in the tub with the typical stance of the Maloriented: fists in front, ready to strike, defending himself from the outside world. Deep down, Thomas was afraid of losing control, of falling apart, of having nothing to do, of dying alone.

Suspecting that Thomas was afraid of intimacy and would probably recoil from any expression of emotion, John Dawes kept his voice level, matter-of-fact. "What do you *hate the most* when people butt into your affairs?" John asked, hoping to help Mr. Konig express himself, so that his anxiety would lessen as he felt validated.

"Damn! When they tell me what to do, boss me around."

His anger out, Tom's voice was not quite so loud. He lowered his fists. His muscles began to relax.

"Did that ever bother you before?" John asked encouraging Mr. Konig to reminisce, to think about a happier time, when he was in control.

"Hell, no! The captain knows how to steer a straight course. You have to take orders on a ship."

John handed Thomas a towel. The old man accepted the towel as a gift and stepped from the tub, drying himself as he recalled the past.

John tried another Validation technique by asking Thomas to imagine the opposite. "Was there ever a time when things went wrong? When someone made a mistake?" he asked.

Tom chuckled, snapping the towel. "That was something. It was me. I got drunk and loaded the wrong cargo. We were stranded in the North Sea with a load of lettuce instead of lobster. Lost my lieutenant stripes."

John Dawes nodded with empathy. "Did you give up the ship? Did you tell the captain to go to hell?"

"Hell, no!" Thomas shot back.

John was trying to help Tom find a familiar coping strategy to overcome present-day losses. "What did you do that time, Mr. Konig?"

"I told the captain I was drunk and I made a mistake and that I'd take my punishment like a man, but I never apologized. I'm not going to take anything back. I'm not going to tell old lady Waters I'm sorry, if that's what you want me to do."

Respecting Thomas' defensive shield, the veteran police officer reassured him, helping the old man hold on to his dignity. "You don't have to apologize to anybody, but do you think that you could swim at the Y instead of in the bathtub? They have a bus that picks you up right outside." The officer knew that the nearby YMCA served seniors well. The next day, the officer would stop by the Y to enlist their help. Thomas might even join the YMCA band instead of banging trash cans in the middle of the night.

"I might do that," said Thomas Konig. He shook hands with the policeman, the emergency medical technicians, and the apartment manager, dismissing them with a wave. He closed the door behind them, forgetting to bolt the double lock.

Thomas Konig remained angry over his losses, but his nocturnal noises stopped. Neighbors complained less, and the police were rarely summoned. He lived in his own apartment until he died.

THE MAILMAN, THE GROCERY CLERK, THE HAIRDRESSER, AND MILLIE STONEWALL

"Poor thing, no mail on her birthday. And she's probably waiting for me in this cold weather at the mailbox." Rudy, the mailman rubbed his aching knee, picturing Millie Stonewall. The thought of her always made his heart ache. Rudy shook his head in wonder. Did Millie remind him of his mother, who also lived alone and was now 85? "Maybe," Rudy reflected, "I worry too much. But then, I can't help it. Poor old thing. Eighty-five years old and living alone on top of that hill—in that big house, with hardly any heat." Rudy imagined Millie, her white hair blowing over her eyes, her food-stained apron flapping with the wind, winding her way down the steep hill to the mailbox, hoping for a letter from her son. Tenaciously, her arthritic fingers would grip the railing her son had finally installed from the house to the street.

"She'll get a big kick out of my birthday card!" Rudy chuckled, his black moustache twitching, anticipating Millie's joyful response. Rudy finished sorting his mail and drove off to deliver Millie's mail.

At that moment, Millie was busy shopping. First in line at the grocery store, she shifted her shopping bag to ease the ache in her shoulder. Bursitis sent flashes of pain through her body. Bravely, Millie Stonewall blinked away the tears, refusing help.

"Please, Mrs. Stonewall, you'll trip on the sidewalk. Let Mike carry it for you." The check-out girl signaled the grocery clerk.

"No, dear. Mike's too busy. I can handle the bag. I'm used to it. It's just my shoulder." Millie's voice dropped to a whisper fraught with agony. She clutched the check-out girl's arm and bent close to her ear to deliver each word. The six people waiting in line leaned forward to catch a stray phrase. "My shoulder hurts so bad that I forgot to get the lettuce. You know how Tweety loves lettuce. She'll be so disappointed. And I won't get to come back for another 3 days because my driveway can't take all that pummeling from my tires. It's a mud driveway, and every time it rains, my driveway disappears. I told Harry before he died to spend the money to put in asphalt, but you remember Harry? My husband? He taught you geography. I think he gave you an *A*. He was a wonderful teacher but a very cheap man. Saving money on a driveway is no saving. Believe me!"

The woman behind Millie could not squelch her mounting irritation. "Please, lady, I have to pick up my son from school, and you're making me very late." The people in line realized that they had been tricked by Millie's urgent whispers. Her social chit-chat began to grate. The people in line began to complain.

"Oh, I'm so sorry. I'll forget the lettuce. But Tweety only eats lettuce." The check-out girl was speechless with frustration. Oblivious, Millie went on. "Do you think he'll try cabbage? I still have a half a head of cabbage. Cabbage looks like lettuce. And his eyes are bad. Canaries have very poor eyesight. I'm sure I read that somewhere. Probably in a nature magazine." Millie turned to confide in the woman behind her, who was becoming more and more frantic thinking of her toddler waiting at nursery school.

"Mrs. Stonewall, why don't you finish checking out while I get the lettuce?" Mike, the 22-year-old grocery clerk, instinctively knew how to validate Millie. His quiet tone reassured her. She paid for her groceries and scurried out the door with Mike. On the way to the car, Mike carried the bag of lettuce, and Millie lugged the rest of her groceries. The young man understood that this old woman had to show the world that she was still strong because she was terrified of losing her strength. He listened gravely as Millie rambled.

"It's not for me, it's for Tweety," she said. "You know, I got that canary to keep me company after Harry died. Harry hated birds: 'Filthy, dirty birds leaving their droppings and God knows what diseases,' Harry used to say. Harry studied rare diseases. He taught geography, did you know that, Mike? I'm sure that he gave you an *A*. You're such a bright boy. Did you know that Harry was a geography teacher in high school?"

"Yes, Mrs. Stonewall. My Dad told me that Mr. Stonewall was a terrific teacher—the best he ever had." Mike knew that 85-year-old Millie was losing her recent memory, often repeating herself without realizing it. He did not expect her to remember, so he did not embarrass her by reminding her of her repetitions. He had learned to admire her storehouse of knowledge and ignore her recent memory loss. When she rambled, frantically moving from one thought to another, Mike understood that she meant to lure him into listening. Millie Stonewall was lonely. The least he could do, thought Mike, was to give her a few quality minutes. The oldest of seven, he was a good listener.

"How come Mr. Stonewall never liked canaries?" he asked, encouraging Millie to express her irritation with her husband.

"Harry got food poisoning from eating a bird. He was never the same after that. He never let me cook a duck, or even a chicken, or anything with feathers. He was sure that he swallowed a feather. That's what did him in. After that, Harry was a very fussy eater. But he always had a delicate stomach, you know, even as a child." Millie patted Mike's cheek, reminiscing about Harry's allergy, her muddy driveway, the chemical composition of feathers, and the benefits of eating lettuce. Satisfied that this young man cared about her, she cheerily waved goodbye and drove off.

Rudy reached Millie's mailbox just as she pulled into her driveway. Vaguely disappointed that she wasn't anxiously waiting for him at her mailbox, or at least trudging down the hill to meet him, Rudy drove up to the house to help her. Millie remembered that Rudy arrived promptly at 3:00 P.M., Tuesday through Saturday. She even remembered the holidays when there was no mail. She timed her grocery shopping accordingly. They got out of their cars and shook hands. Rudy took the groceries out of her car.

"Rudy, you are the sweetest man. But I am perfectly capable of carrying my own groceries. It's just my bursitis

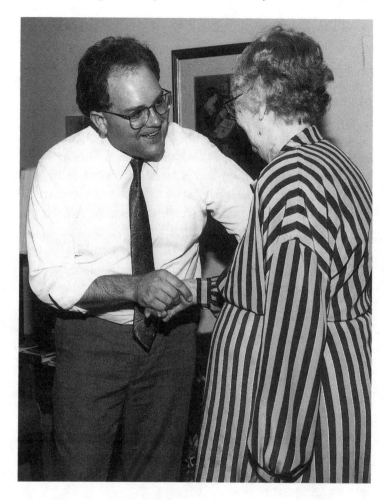

that acts up when I carry too much in one hand. But I can switch hands, and then I'll be fine."

"You're 86 today, Millie. Happy birthday!" Rudy beamed, bending over to kiss Millie's cheek and give her his birthday card.

Millie Stonewall stopped dead in her tracks. She stared at Rudy, her face white. "Rudy, I'm 68, not 86. You're mixed up. Today is not my birthday. My birthday is September 4th, 1906."

"That's right!" Rudy nodded, happily. "And today is September 4, 1992. Look, here's the paper." Rudy showed Millie the headlines, with the date in bold print.

"That's not today's paper. I just read the paper in the supermarket, and those are not the headlines. Rudy, you better see the eye doctor. I think your eyes are not as sharp as they used to be. Harry's eyes started to go when he was about your age. Glaucoma sets in. Harry never listened when I told him to get his pressure checked. No, Harry knew better. Where do you think his diabetes came from? Not from his family. No one in Harry's family ever had diabetes."

Rudy grew quiet. He carried Millie's groceries from her car into her kitchen. With a sudden flash of insight, Rudy saw Millie as she was—an old woman fighting old age; unable to ask for help; fooling herself to keep from falling apart; cleverly manipulating him to help her carry her groceries, read her mail, light her stove, and even chop her wood on weekends. Millie wasn't helpless. She was a survivor.

No one knew Millie better than Rudy's wife, Tessie. Tessie had been Millie's hairdresser for 25 years. That night, Tessie gave her husband a blow-by-blow description of *her* last encounter with the old lady.

"Tessie," Millie had wailed, "you're putting some chemicals in that bottle that take off my hair. Look, Tessie! This whole side is getting bald. I had a full head of hair when I walked in here." Millie squinted, her nose pressed to the mirror, to show Tessie her bald spots. "I always had beautiful hair. My crowning glory, Harry used to say. You know what that means, Tessie? Crowning glory? That means I always had a lot of hair. Those chemicals are taking it out, little by little."

Tessie understood Validation. She knew not to argue with Millie. She knew that Millie was afraid of losing her hair. When Millie asked about getting a wig, Tessie rephrased Millie's words. "Do you think that some chemicals are taking out your hair?"

Mollified, Millie nodded. Tessie then used polarity. "Which side do you think is the worst? The right side or the left side?"

"The right side," responded Millie, peering closer to the mirror, squinting her eyes, adjusting her trifocals, then frowning. "No. The left side. The left side is the worst. What are we going to do, Tessie? Can you get a different shampoo?"

Tessie reminisced. "What kind of shampoo did we use when your hair was not falling out? Do you remember, Millie?"

"I think it was that yellow bottle. The one with the conditioner in it. But I don't think they make that anymore. That was almost 10 years ago, remember, when Harry was still alive?"

"What color was your hair then? Was it blonde or light brown? Did Harry like it blonde?" Tessie continued to explore the past, knowing that Millie missed her husband more than she missed her hair. She needed to grieve to keep on going.

Millie would continue to complain, to whine, to manipulate her neighbors. Her memory loss worsened, but people in the community like Rudy, Mike, and Tessie helped her to continue to live independently, in her own home. Their sensitivity kept her fighting spirit alive. She died 6 years later, at 92.

THE DOCTOR, THE MEALS ON
WHEELS VOLUNTEER, AND SAMUEL GOODE

"Kindly remove yourself from my icebox, old woman." Samuel Goode, J.D., former professor of law, spoke stiffly, his husky voice clipped, his plaid bow tie quivering. The recipient of his subdued hostility, Maureen O'Connell, a 63-year-old novice volunteer for the Meals on Wheels program, shrank, almost disappearing into the refrigerator.

"But, Mr. Goode, everything in here is spoiled." Her muffled voice found its way from her throat to Sam Goode's good ear. "You'll die of food poisoning if you drink that milk. It's 6 months old! And your meat smells terrible. The eggs are all rotten. . . ."

In his curt courthouse voice, Samuel Goode informed Maureen, "I am *Professor* Goode, and my eggs are not rotten. That is an unfounded accusation. You are smelling your body odor. Old women notoriously give off a pungent stench. Moreover, Madam, you are trespassing. Have the courtesy to remove yourself from my premises. I am a powerful attorney in this town, and I can have you incarcerated, just like that!" Sam Goode tried to snap his arthritic fingers. It was a futile, soundless attempt, but it bore the mark of authority.

Maureen O'Connell would not give up. Her husband had ended his life in a nursing home, and Maureen couldn't forgive herself. To make amends, she was dedicating her retirement to helping old people like this 88-year-old man stay in their own homes. Poking her gray hair into the refrigerator, Maureen pulled out six smelly, rotten eggs, holding each one under Sam's nose for inspection. With utter disdain, Sam flared his nostrils, turned his back on Maureen and the eggs, and picked up the telephone to dial.

"Professor Samuel Goode here, Sergeant. There's an insane woman harassing me. I want her out of my offices within 3 minutes or I will press charges." Sam Goode did not wait for the policeman to reply. He cradled the telephone quietly and folded his hands. His eyes shot Maureen a warning. She blanched, but stood her ground, dropping the smelly eggs into the garbage. He began to pace, his bushy white mustache bristling. "I will wait you out, Madam. You are about to be punished." Samuel Goode unclasped his hands to reach for his cane.

Maureen had had many years of experience in dodging her late husband's cane. Hastily, she stuck her black felt hat on her head and bolted from Sam Goode's house.

"I can't go back there. I'm so sorry," Maureen nearly wept, apologizing to the Meals on Wheels volunteer coordinator. "The man terrifies me. He'll hit me if I go back, just like my husband used to do. And he refuses to eat our meals. He tosses everything in the fridge and forgets that he put it there. His neighbors told me that he eats out once a day at the Chinese restaurant. If you ask me, Samuel Goode has Alzheimer's disease."

The coordinator called the social worker from the Department of Health and Human Services. She referred Sam Goode to a neurologist, Dr. Alan Farley, who administered a battery of medical, laboratory, neurological, and psychological tests—a complete diagnostic workup for a case of dementia.

"Son, I appreciate that you're doing an excellent job with those test questions." Sam Goode patronizingly patted the 43-year-old neurologist's shoulder. "But, young man, don't you think you should find out the president's name by *yourself*? I'm not going to tell you. Just read today's paper. His name'll be in there somewhere. Young people have lost their initiative. That is a sad fact."

Al Farley grinned, valuing the old man's intuitive wisdom. Subconsciously, on a deep level of awareness, Sam Goode knew that he could not perform adequately and would not risk taking the test. Dr. Farley had insight into the psyche, not only into the brain. He understood Validation theory and applied it in his practice. He realized that this once brilliant attorney was denying his recent memory loss in order to maintain his self-respect. This old man was a master confabulator. Sam Goode could not and would not answer the questions on the Wechsler Memory Scale test, or on any other dementia scale test. When Dr. Farley asked Sam to count backward from 10, the old man replied, "Son, if you're going to be a doctor, you better bone up on your mathematics."

Dr. Farley tried again. "You were an attorney, weren't you, Professor Goode? And you also taught law?"

"Still do!" Sam Goode shot back. "And I expect that I could teach you a thing or two."

"I know that you could," Dr. Farley agreed, emphatically. "Where do you live now, Professor Goode?" Al called Sam Goode by his last name. Addressing Sam by his first name would be disrespectful.

Sam had forgotten his address, so he answered quickly. "With my mother. She's an old lady. My father's dead. I've never been married, so we kind of take care of each other."

"Professor Goode," Dr. Farley tried reality orientation to determine the extent of the disorientation, "you know that you are now 88 years old. Your mother is no longer alive."

"She's alive on a technicality!" Sam explained patiently.

"How old would you say you are?" Dr. Farley asked.

"Over 30," Sam said coyly.

"Do you think you could be 88?" he asked.

"Well . . . " Sam Goode rubbed his mustache thoughtfully, his brow wrinkling. "I could do the work of 88 people, but I wouldn't say that I'm 88 years old."

Respectfully, Dr. Farley rephrased Sam Goode's words. "You can do the work of 88 people?"

"Not at one time, you understand." Sam Goode was beginning to trust this young doctor. Even though Sam was deaf in one ear, he heard the respect in Dr. Farley's voice. "Young man, you've got old chairs. My rump is getting stiff from sitting so long." Sam pulled himself up from the leather chair and began pacing.

"Will you read this story, Professor Goode, and give me your opinion?" Al wanted to try another psychological comprehension test. His trifocals perched on the tip of his nose, Sam Goode peered at the paper, pacing all the while. Dr. Farley waited patiently. Suddenly, Sam straightened his spine, cleared his throat, and shoved the paper under the doctor's nose.

"Sir, this brief is resplendent with resolutions that have no bearing on the credibility of the witness. These paragraphs are absolutely irrelevant. I move that we dispense with these inane formalities. Let us move to the proper closure of the case, with, of course, preparations for future contacts."

"I hear you loud and clear," said Dr. Farley, who had been listening closely. "Are you telling me that these tests have no bearing on your case?" Sam Goode smiled and nodded. Dr. Farley became thoughtful. "The tests are irrelevant because they don't measure your wisdom."

"Son, I told you I'd teach you a thing or two." Sam was immensely pleased with himself. He added grudgingly, "But, you're a fast learner. Gotta give you credit!"

"Professor Goode, your students were lucky. Would you object to future contacts with someone who could benefit from your knowledge?"

"I never had any children," said Sam. "Too busy becoming a topnotch attorney. I wouldn't mind a young person around, now and then." Uncomfortable with his yearning, Sam's eyes shifted to the floor. Dr. Farley nodded with empathy. In Time Confusion, Sam's controls were beginning to loosen. His emotions needed to be released. Sam Goode needed a validating caregiver whom he could trust, someone with whom he could reminisce and express his fears and unfulfilled desires. A validating relationship could prevent Professor Goode from withdrawing inward to Repetitive Motion. With Validation, he would be communicating until he died.

"Professor Goode, I probably won't be seeing you for some time, but I have a colleague who could learn a lot from you. Would you be willing to see that person on a regular basis?" Dr. Farley's voice was matter-of-fact, full of genuine respect.

"No objection," Sam Goode's voice vibrated. The two men shook hands. Professor Goode strode out straight and tall.

Every Friday, from 3:00 to 5:00 P.M., Sam reminisced with a social worker trained in Validation. Together, they reviewed his triumphs and his defeats. They chuckled at judges, sneered at opposing attorneys, marveled at Sam Goode's accomplishments. Professor Goode no longer stashed rotten eggs in his refrigerator. Reluctantly, he accepted food from the new Meals on Wheels volunteer. He died at age 91, in his own home.

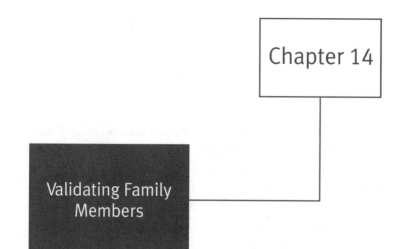

Chapter 14

Validating Family
Members

ANN AND HER MOTHER, TRUDY

The telephone rings for the tenth time in the last hour. Ann, 56, wearily picks up the receiver, knowing full well that it's her mother, Trudy, 82. "Ann, where are you? I've been all alone and the Meals on Wheels people haven't come. They should have been here hours ago. There's nothing in the house. I can't go out to go shopping because then I might miss them. Can't you come over and..."

"Mom, it's 10 in the morning. The Meals on Wheels people come around noon. You should have gone to the community center this morning. I told you. You've called me 10 times in the last hour. You're just bored."

"What do you mean it's 10 o'clock, my clock says it's 2 in the afternoon. Have all my clocks stopped working?

Oh, God. Who's going to fix them? I'll miss all my appointments. I'll be lost..." and crying, she hangs up on Ann.
Ann sets down the receiver, frustrated and furious. Her mother always does this. If it's not one thing, it's another—anything to get Ann to come over and take care of her. She's always done that her whole life. Whenever there was something wrong, Trudy called Ann, and Ann would come fix it. In the past, that happened once in a while, and Ann was usually pleased to be able to help her mother out. These days, Trudy calls every day, making things up just to get Ann to come to her house. Ann has a family of her own, a husband and three children who need her as well, not to mention a full-time job. Ann also feels helpless and doesn't know what to do. The current situation can't go on for much longer and the only thing Ann can think of is to place her mother in a protected living situation.

Validating a close relative is different from validating a friend, a client, or a stranger. Family relationships are complex and filled with emotional pitfalls. Patterns of behavior that were developed early in the relationship continue even when they don't necessarily fit or work. In the previous story, Ann is stuck in her role as "fixer-upper." When her mother calls for help, her first reaction is to fix the situation, whatever it is. It's a pattern that began very early on in the mother–daughter relationship. When Ann's dad left the family, Trudy turned to her when she had to make big decisions. Even as a little girl, Ann helped shoulder the responsibilities of her mother. Later, when Trudy's sister died, Ann made all the funeral arrangements. She wanted to help her mother and knew that Trudy really couldn't handle it all. Now the pattern is set: Trudy can't handle things, and Ann reacts by taking over and fixing the situation.

Here are other typical examples of patterns that are played out between family members and disoriented elderly people:

- A mother who can't let go of the mothering role and calls her son every day to see how he's doing and check up on him.

- A husband who has always depended on his wife to take care of the house and prepare his meals, now that his wife is disoriented and he can no longer do those things, he gets angry at her for letting him down.

- A father who always wanted his children to be curious and learn about new things, now clips articles out of newspapers and magazines every day and sends packets to his children. The son, tired of this constant pressure, throws the packets away without even opening them.

Validating a disoriented relative is difficult for a number of reasons:

- Both individuals are acting and reacting based on a long history together. See the previous examples.

- The oriented person often expects the disoriented relative to be like he or she always "was." "My mother doesn't swear like that."

- The oriented person expects his or her relative to behave "normally" or is embarrassed that he or she does not behave normally. "Stop acting crazy. Why can't you be normal?"

- The oriented person feels angry, disappointed, or helpless because of the disorientation; doesn't understand it; or doesn't know what to do. "It's no use visiting my father, he doesn't talk to me."

- The oriented person often feels rejected when he or she is not recognized by the disoriented person. "My husband doesn't even know who I am. You know he locked me out of the house thinking I was some stranger."

- The oriented person often feels scared that it could happen to him or her. "Will I become crazy like my father?"

- The oriented person often feels guilty about the disoriented relative. "I should have been there more often."

- The oriented person is often financially burdened by the disoriented relative. "How am I going to pay for the help my mother needs?"

Validating means accepting the relative exactly as he or she is in the moment, not judging him or her, and understanding that there is a good reason underlying the disoriented behavior. The oriented person needs to face the loss of the parent or partner he or she once knew. It's important for the person who wants to validate to acknowledge the anger, disappointment, or helplessness he or she feels, and to express those feelings with someone who listens, but not with the disoriented relative. Feelings of anger, disappointment, and frustration about the situation hamper communication with disoriented relatives. They cannot respond to your feelings in a way that will make you feel better.

TIPS FOR FAMILY MEMBERS WHO
WANT TO VALIDATE DISORIENTED RELATIVES

In addition to all of the techniques that you have read about, here are some special tips, or variations of techniques, that might help you communicate with your disoriented relative.

- Centering is key. You can't validate if you are filled with your own anger, frustration, or disappointment. First, you must "shelve," or put aside, your feelings in order to have empathy. Breathing exercises, creative visualization, and meditation are all good ways of setting aside your feelings for the moment that you are validating. It is equally important to take your feelings "off the shelf" once you are finished validating.

- The best way to observe the disoriented relative is technically—in order to gain some emotional distance. Is the voice harsh? Is the breathing rapid? Is the upper lip tensed and pursed? Go through a mental checklist. Calibrate all of the changes and signals that you can pick up. Now you can recognize the feelings, symbols, and issues that are important to the disoriented person in the moment.

- Try to recognize the triggers in your relationship. What issues from the past remind you of the present situation? Ask yourself, "When did that happen before?" Try to recognize and be aware so that you don't get hooked in old patterns.

- The verbal Validation techniques of rephrasing and polarity are particularly useful. Remember to rephrase with empathy and energy. Sometimes reminiscing together about a shared experience can feel good. Talking about times when the disoriented person could function might help bring back some of those dormant abilities. For example, "Remember, Mom, when Dad went away to Japan for a month and you had to take care of everything? How did you handle that?"

- Find familiar music or songs to sing, play, or hum together. Even nonverbal, disoriented older adults respond to music.

- Try to find two techniques that work often. Practice those until you don't have to think about them and you can use them appropriately and easily.

- Remember, always try to respond first to the needs of the disoriented person, rather than react from your own needs.

ANN AND TRUDY—WITH VALIDATION

The telephone rings for the third time in the last hour. Ann takes a deep breath as she picks up the receiver, knowing full well that it's her mother. "Ann, where are you? I've been all alone, and the Meals on Wheels people haven't come. They should have been here hours ago. There's nothing in the house. I can't go out to go shopping because then I might miss them. Can't you come over and ..."

As she was listening to her mother, Ann heard her mother's voice was high pitched and tight. Trudy was speaking rapidly and her breathing sounded quick and shallow. Matching her mother's voice tone, Ann answered, "Mom, where do you think the Meals on Wheels people could be?"

Trudy, speaking slightly slower and a touch deeper, "Uh, I don't know. They usually are right on time. There's that nice girl who always spends a few extra minutes talking with me."

Ann responds, modulating her voice lower, "What do you like to talk about with her?"

"Oh, we talk about our children. She's got three kids all in school. She likes to look at my pictures of you kids when you were young."

"Do you miss those times?"

"Ach, Annie. Sometimes it's so lonely being old."

"How about coming over for dinner this Sunday and bringing those old pictures. I bet my three would love to see those."

"Can you really handle having me over? I don't want to be a burden?"

"Yes, Mom. It would be a pleasure. Shall I have Ben pick you up at 6?"

"That would be fine. Well, I've got to go now. My program comes on at 11. See you Sunday."

"Bye Mom. Love you."

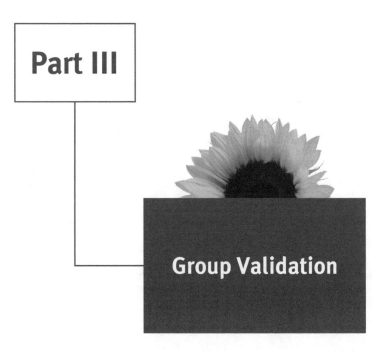

Part III

Group Validation

The use of Validation as a method of communicating with disoriented old-old people originated in 1963 in *group* settings. Some disoriented old-old people may derive more benefit from participating in a Validation group than from individual Validation therapy. Validation groups can be formed in a variety of settings, including nursing homes, adult day care centers, small group homes, senior centers, and private homes. Groups can be led by professionals or by volunteers trained in Validation.

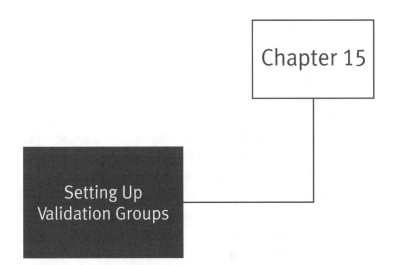

Chapter 15

Setting Up
Validation Groups

THE VALUE OF A VALIDATION GROUP

Sometimes a group can be even more effective than a one-to-one relationship with old-old people who are in Time Confusion and Repetitive Motion because:

- A group produces energy, preventing withdrawal.

- A group heightens attention span. Disoriented old-old people have difficulty in concentrating and are losing speech. Therefore, one-to-one relationships can last for only 5–15 minutes, whereas a Validation group often lasts for 1 hour, during which time individuals interact with each other.

- A group helps participants solve problems and care about each other.

- A group gives participants the opportunity to restore familiar social and work roles and family relationships.

- Moving, singing, touching, talking, problem-solving, produces group cohesion. Withdrawal turns to involvement. The group develops a rhythm: a beginning, with anticipation; a middle, which engages group members in a common purpose; and an end, which looks forward to the next meeting.

- In a group, participants express themselves verbally and nonverbally. Often, the group stimulates social controls. Disoriented old-old people become motivated to control negative behaviors (e.g., pacing, pounding, swearing) as they regain dignity in the Validation group.

- A group helps participants restore a sense of worth because they are listened to and respected by others in the Validation group. They regain independence as they perform their group roles.

The goals of a Validation group are:

1. To stimulate interaction

2. To encourage participants to take on social roles

3. To generate a sense of well-being and happiness

4. To develop social controls

5. To increase verbal behaviors (Feil, 1992b)

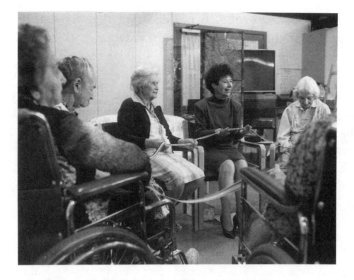

WHO BENEFITS FROM GROUP VALIDATION?

The selection of group members is crucial to the success of the Validation group. Maloriented people who are afraid of feelings and terrified of losing their recent memory and social controls do not belong in a Validation group, where feelings are freely expressed and group members often do not conform to social rules. Maloriented people can benefit from a *reality-type group* that does not stress the importance of knowing the present day or date. *Task-oriented groups* that do not stress feelings—such as a current events group; a resident's council that recommends changes in food or management of the facility; a baking, painting, music, or flower-arranging group; a Remotivation group; a Reminiscing group that does not dwell on emotions—may benefit a Maloriented person.

Before the group, it is important that the caregiver build trust through one-to-one Validation with the Maloriented. The Maloriented person who is a blamer can alienate peers. The caregiver must often limit the Maloriented person in order to preserve relationships. If the Maloriented person trusts the caregiver, he or she will save any complaints for the individual Validation sessions. Maloriented people often enjoy a role as the caregiver's assistant in the Validation Group, but never as a group member.

People who should not be included in a Validation group are:

- Maloriented people who fear disorientation
- People with a history of psychotic illness
- People who are oriented, but with a chronic illness, such as aphasia after a stroke
- People with Parkinson's disease without dementia
- People with cognitive disabilities
- People with early-onset Alzheimer's disease who act out aggressively and who pace during a group meeting
- People in Repetitive Motion and Vegetation who need individual Validation, not group Validation
- Time Confused people who have never belonged to groups and who are uncomfortable in a group setting (e.g., a former farmer who has never socialized or verbalized will be uncomfortable in a Validation group; he needs individual Validation.)

The group should include at least six people in Time Confusion and one or two in Repetitive Motion, providing that they will sit and remain in the group. Touch by the caregiver or other nurturing group members often reassures the person in Repetitive Motion, who will stop pacing and begin relating to others in the Validation group. There is little energy produced with less than six people, making it difficult for the worker to elicit verbal and nonverbal interactions. However, if the facility has few residents who are in Time Confusion, then no more than four people in Repetitive Motion should be included in the Validation group. In this case, there is little verbal interaction, but mainly singing and movement.

The group should include at least two or three people in Time Confusion who are verbal and who have experience with leadership roles, such as a mother with many children, a businessman, or a church leader. Men as well as women should be included in the Validation group to stimulate energy, which often stimulates dormant speech. It is important that groups meet once each week. If members do not meet regularly, they soon regress.

THE ROLE OF THE VALIDATION GROUP WORKER

The role of the Validation group worker is to:

1. Provide privacy. Disoriented old-old people need a private place to meet, without interruptions.

2. Coordinate staff support and the necessary materials for each meeting. The worker provides regular in-services to staff, presenting Validation goals and results.

3. Provide security. Disoriented old-old people must feel that they will not be hurt by abusive peers or peers who create anxiety. Many Maloriented people, psychotic elderly people, and people with early-onset Alzheimer's disease often strike out without provocation. These people should not be included in a Validation group. People in Repetitive Motion who constantly pace or moan may not benefit from group Validation and may keep other group members from feeling secure.

4. Facilitate interaction between group members.

5. Give group members an opportunity to solve problems by stating simply, using one-syllable words, two alternatives to a problem that disoriented old-old can solve (e.g., "When you miss someone you love, should you cry by yourself or find a friend?"). Wise, intuitive old-old people can solve universal problems (e.g., how to find love, how to restore self-worth, how to express human emotions).

6. Give familiar social roles to each group member. These roles should restore well-being and not raise anxiety. The roles must be easy to perform.

7. Provide a structure. Disoriented old-old people feel safe in a familiar place. They need a group ritual. The group has a beginning, middle, and end. The Validation worker helps group members move from the beginning to the end through the group ritual.

8. Link the behavior of the old-old person to his or her human needs by asking group members to help each other. A woman rocks, holding her hand as if it were her baby. She strokes the hand-baby. The Validation

group worker relates the woman's behavior to her need to be a mother. The worker asks group members how to help the woman restore motherhood, eliciting group interactions. Group members rally around the woman, wanting to help her.

9. Observe the emotions of group members.

10. State their emotion and match the emotion, tying together similar emotions. Disoriented old-old people will express their emotions verbally, with touch, and with eye contact. Expressing common emotions links the group together, creating a "we" feeling. Group members begin to feel a sense of belonging.

11. Use ambiguity when disoriented old-old people can no longer use dictionary words. The Validation worker is able to communicate even when disoriented old-old cannot explain what they mean. A group member says, "That mentalink is okay with the substantial miterlucks." The group member is smiling, pointing to his brain. The worker rephrases, making sense of the unique word combinations, using vague pronouns (e.g., "it," "we," "someone," "something") to fill in for the nondictionary words. "Do you mean that mentally we have luck with it?"

12. Use the Validation techniques for the Time Confused and for people in Repetitive Motion to elicit interactions between members (see pages 80–85 and pages 94–97).

13. For all group members, learn about their past relationships, find out which songs are familiar to them, figure out their movement potential, and learn about their

social and work history so that you can engage group members in common themes and solve common emotional problems.

14. Use touch and genuine, focused eye contact, music, and rhythms with each group member to stimulate nonverbal interactions.

15. Evaluate progress with co-workers.

16. Involve families through regular family workshops, teaching relatives the Validation techniques. Families often enjoy volunteering, helping the professional caregiver with music during special celebrations in the Validation group, such as holidays and birthday parties.

17. Prepare a topic with a universal problem to solve, but be willing to abandon it if a group member presents a different problem. For example, a group member wails suddenly. The worker asks the group to help this person feel better and explores the sudden sorrow of the group member.

THE ROLE OF THE VALIDATION GROUP CO-WORKER

A Validation group co-worker is a second caregiver who helps with movements, wheelchair dancing, transportation, and the evaluation of progress. The caregiver is often so focused on one or two individuals that he or she does not notice interactions by other group members. The co-worker is an observer who can give feedback after the meeting. The validating caregiver and the co-worker should meet after each meeting to evaluate progress by completing the Validation group evaluation form (Figure 3). The caregiver and

Name	Talks in group	Makes eye contact	Touches	Smiles	Shows leadership	Participates	
							Date:
							General comments on group meetings:
							Conflicts:
							Plans for next week:

0—Never does   1—Rarely does   2—Occasionally does   3—Frequently does   4—Always does

Figure 3. Validation group evaluation form. The group worker and co-worker can work together to complete the evaluation after each group meeting.

co-worker can exchange roles. However, there can be only one main, nurturing caregiver during a meeting, as disoriented old-old people cannot relate to two people at the same time in a Validation group.

ESTABLISHING A VALIDATION GROUP

Step 1: Gathering Information and Selecting Group Members

The caregiver must observe the physical characteristics of potential group members to assess their stage of orientation or disorientation. Caregivers should remember that old-old people do not stay in one stage, but can move from Malorientation to Repetitive Motion within a 5-minute period. However, the person usually is in one stage most of the time. The caregiver must meet with a potential group member at different times of the day for at least 15 minutes each time, over a period of several weeks in order to assess the stage of disorientation. For example, old-old people change their behaviors at night, when fears of abandonment reoccur. Maloriented people often become Time Confused in their search for parental love.

The caregiver must observe the potential group member's psychological characteristics and interview the person, using the techniques for the Maloriented and Time Confused presented in Part I. For example, if old-old people do not want to be touched, they are usually oriented or Maloriented, and do not belong in a Validation group. If they know present time and place, the role of the caregiver, and the names of their children, then they are too oriented to benefit from a Validation group. The following "here and now" questions can help in assessing potential group participants:

1. How do you like this home?

2. Have you been here a long time?

3. Do you like your roommate?

4. Is the food cooked enough? Is it hot enough?

5. Do you have to wait a long time to be served?

6. How do you like the other people?

7. Do you have enough to do here in this home?

8. Do you like the nurses?

9. How often do you see the doctor here?

10. What do you do during the day?

Oriented or Maloriented old-old people will answer these questions appropriately. Disoriented old-old people will either bring up another subject, be unable to answer with dictionary words, or will restore the past to present time. For example, when asked "Do you like the other people?" a disoriented old-old person might respond, "Oh—they are my dear friends. I've known that woman for yarlongs. We went to church together, in Simelfat."

The following "there and then" questions can also help in assessing the stage of the old-old individual:

1. Where were you born?

2. What work did you do?

3. Are you married?

4. What did your spouse do? What did your father do?

5. How long did you live in this city?

6. Did you live in a big house?

7. Do you have sisters and brothers?

8. Did you help take care of your sisters and brothers?

9. What religion are you?

10. Did you sing in church?

11. What do you do for fun? Sing? Dance? Participate in a social club?

The Time Confused person may respond, "I still work. My mother is still alive. I have to take care of the children." The caregiver can discover the appropriate group role and the goal of a particular individual by asking questions that explore the past. For example, if a person reveals that he or she has always liked to sing, the caregiver can give that person the role of song leader in the group.

In addition to assessing the stage of potential group members, "here and now" and "there and then" questions will provide the caregiver with information necessary to conduct a Validation group:

- What social role is familiar and comfortable to this person?

- What is the goal of group Validation for this person (e.g., prevent withdrawal to Repetitive Motion; increase verbal behaviors; increase eye contact; increase nonverbal interactions; increase energy; decrease crying, pacing, moaning)?

- What stage is this person in most of the time?

- What topic or unresolved issue will engage this person (e.g., unexpressed grief at the death of a child, an unhappy marriage, loss of a spouse, loss of a beloved parent, loneliness, boredom, the need to be active and to be working, anger at a parent or a sibling)?

- Does the person respond to music? If so, to which songs? The caregiver, knowing that Time Confused people cannot identify song titles or remember how the song begins, must start singing the familiar song. Familiar melodies often return when simulated by the worker, however, and Time Confused people and those in Repetitive Motion will often join the caregiver and sing each word.

- What is the person's capacity for movement? Can he or she bear weight? What is his or her medical history?

- Whom can this person relate to? To a woman? To a man? Knowing past relationships can help the caregiver know where to seat this person in the group. Time Confused people and those in Repetitive motion cannot see or hear well. They will relate to the person next to them, not to the person opposite them. The worker should seat people next to each other who have a positive potential relationship.

Step 2: Involving Staff

Individual Validation can be implemented without the support of all departments, but a worker cannot successfully conduct the Validation group without the involvement of all levels of staff. Key staff must assist the worker with:

1. Transporting residents who are in wheelchairs

2. Toileting residents before the Validation group

3. Securing a private room

4. Ensuring privacy (e.g., staff should not interrupt the meeting and take out group members)

5. Ensuring that residents are not sedated before the meeting

6. Suggesting new members when group members die or when the group is ready to incorporate a new member

7. Informing the validating caregiver about group members' behaviors

8. Informing the validating caregiver about family relationships

9. Suggesting new topics

10. Evaluating progress on a monthly basis

11. Informing the Validation caregiver about relationships between group members outside the meeting

For example, in a staff meeting, the occupational therapist (OT) might inform the validating caregiver that Wednesdays are OT days for three of the proposed group members. The Validation group should not be scheduled to meet on Wednesdays because group members would be too tired after the OT session. Another example of staff involvement could be the social worker suggesting a new member who will be suitable for the Validation group. Or perhaps the director of volunteers may suggest a volunteer who could help the validating caregiver with the music portion of the group.

Step 3: Establishing Goals and Assigning Roles

From the people selected for the Validation Group, the worker must choose:

- One Time Confused person with leadership ability (e.g., a former head of a club, a former business-person) who can begin and end the group meetings
- Four or five people in Time Confusion who enjoy talking, singing, and relating to others. An individual with early-onset Alzheimer's disease whose behavior is predictable and who enjoys being nurtured by wise disoriented old-old people can benefit from the Validation group. A Maloriented person can become the caregiver's assistant.
- One or two people in Repetitive Motion who will respond immediately to the worker's touch, and whose repetitive movements will cease when they are validated

Roles give structure to the meetings and help individuals participate. They remain the same for the life of the group.

The caregiver assigns roles that match the background of each individual. For example, the caregiver must find a song leader who enjoys singing, such as a former choir member; a hostess or host who can serve refreshments; and a movement leader who can lead the dancing or rhythm band that energizes the group. Possible group roles include the following:

- Welcomer, or chairperson, who opens and closes the meeting
- Song leader, rhythm leader, or bandleader
- Poetry reader
- Prayer leader (e.g., a former rabbi or minister)
- Chair arranger (e.g., a former architect or builder)
- Flower arranger (e.g., a former gardener)
- Emotional leader (e.g., a nurturing old-old person who enjoys solving other people's problems)

The same role should be maintained throughout the life of the group. With the security of performing the same role week after week, old-old people become more and more eloquent, their roles are performed more smoothly, and they regain dignity.

Roles can be created to suit the needs of the individual. A person who hums becomes the song leader. A person who pounds and tells everyone to "shut up" can become the group's "shutter-upper." This person opens and closes the meeting with a gavel, gaining everyone's respect. This individual will no longer yell "shut up" inappropriately— the need for respect and control will have been validated. Men who act out sexually become the dance leaders, touching women in socially acceptable ways. Their sexual acting out will lessen outside the group meetings because their needs will have been validated in the group, where social controls are tapped, and group members help each other express their feelings in socially acceptable ways.

Sometimes, former roles create anxiety. A former concert pianist may tremble when she sits in front of the piano, unable to play, fearful of failure. A former secretary may not want to take the minutes of the meetings because she was fired at age 65 when she could no longer take short-hand. As soon as she has a pad and pencil, she remembers her feelings of shame. This woman could become a song leader, if she enjoys singing. If the caregiver makes a mistake and assigns the wrong role, the Time Confused person will not remember and will quickly assume a role that does not create anxiety, providing the caregiver is always nurturing and respectful. Time Confused people and those in Repetitive Motion will forgive mistakes, because they intuitively know that the caregiver cares for and respects them.

Sometimes an individual cannot perform a social role in the group, but enjoys listening and offering an occasional opinion. This person benefits from the group without a role.

Step 4: Planning the Content of the Meeting

Music, movement, talk, and sharing food are the ingredients of a Validation group. The amount of time spent on each ingredient depends on the capacity of group members during the meeting. Each group meeting varies. Energy levels, moods, verbal and nonverbal behaviors fluctuate during the day. The validating caregiver moves with the rhythm of the group. Although each meeting is different, the caregiver follows the same ritual, or order of events, to give feelings of security to group members. All group members know that the nurturing caregiver will ensure their well-being during the meeting, all feel comfortable expressing themselves through music, movement, talk, eye contact, and eating together.

Music

Music stimulates verbal interactions and energy. The caregiver must know love songs, lullabies, marching songs, happy songs, and sad songs that are familiar to the group members. (Songs that are familiar to disoriented old-old people include: "Let Me Call You Sweetheart," "Daisy," "You Are My Sunshine," "When Johnny Comes Marching Home," "When Irish Eyes Are Smiling," "You Take the High Road," Army and Navy songs from World War II, and "I Want a Girl.") Each kind of song should be used to match the topic and the mood of the group. Group members who cannot express their feelings with words can sing their emotions. A marching song can help the group express common feelings of anger; a love song frees sexual feelings and memories of a spouse; a lullaby stimulates memories of mother and motherhood. Group members often enjoy using rhythm band instruments, such as bells and cymbals, when they sing. This often stimulates Repetitive Movers to interact in the group. Verbal behaviors sometime occur after movement and singing. Movement and songs end the meeting on an up beat, and group members will look forward to the next meeting with positive anticipation.

Movement

Movement activities represent an important element of the Validation group, and are crucial to encouraging interaction among participants. Some simple equipment is useful:

- A soft ball, large enough to be held comfortably in two hands when the fingers are curled, can be passed from one participant to the next to stimulate interaction.

- A bean bag can be thrown about by group members, helping them rid themselves of angry feelings.

- A large rubber band can be grasped by group members as they dance to release tension.

- Scarves can be used for dancing and swaying to the music. Moving scarves to the beat of the music, tapping the feet, square dancing, circle dancing (e.g., "The Hokey Pokey")—all of these activities create joy, heighten energy, and give the group a feeling of togetherness and well-being. People in wheelchairs need not be excluded, as they can also sway to the music.

Arts and craft projects, finger painting, kneading dough, using puppets, rhythm band, and gardening are suggestions for movement activities. The occupational therapist, music therapist, art therapist, and dance therapist can help with appropriate movements and songs that will not increase anxiety for disoriented old-old people.

The validating caregiver must not offer activities that are too difficult for disoriented old-old individuals. They no longer have good eyesight, cognitive capacity, or the energy and motivation needed to perform complicated physical tasks. The movement, music, and talk must conform to the capacities of group members.

Topics for Discussion

Some verbal interactions are vital in the Validation group to stimulate dormant brain functions. Very often, disoriented old-old people will talk in the Validation group for the first time in months. Topics should relate to emotions and unmet human needs such as love, belonging, the search for meaning and identity, the need to be active and useful, and the need to express emotions and to be heard by a trusted other.

Some specific suggested topics for group meetings include:

1. Do you miss your parents?

2. Do you miss your home?

3. Do you miss your job?

4. Do you feel bored?

5. Are you afraid of being alone?

6. What makes a person happy?

7. What makes a person sad?

8. How does one find meaning in life?

9. How did you get along with your sisters or brothers?

10. What do you love most about your mother or father?

11. What do you love most about your husband or wife?

12. What are the qualities of a good friend?

13. How do you get along with "crazy" people?

14. What is "crazy?"

15. What makes people act the way they do?

16. What happens when a person gets old?

17. What do you do when you miss your spouse?

18. Should we prepare to die?

Refreshments

Eating in a social setting is nurturing for all participants and provides a role for the host or hostess. What is served depends upon the culture of the members of the group. Whatever is served, it must be carefully selected, so that the group members can eat easily and not spill. Plates must be lightweight and easy to pass, so that the host or hostess is not embarrassed by spilling. The validating caregiver must also consult with the dietician on selecting refreshments that are appropriate for the participants. Food must be prepared beforehand, so that the Time Confused host or hostess can easily pass the plate of cookies, serve the drinks, and pass the napkins. Performing this role is important to the host or hostess, who will feel a sense of renewed self-esteem. Someone in Repetitive Motion, who likes to pat, can be the napkin passer.

Step 5: Preparing the Room

The caregiver should prepare the meeting room, arranging the chairs so that potential friends will sit next to each other. A table should not be used. A table separates individuals and makes it difficult for them to see, hear, or touch each other. A table can be used later, during refreshments or during an activity such as finger painting, gardening, or kneading dough. The validating caregiver should seat the group members in a circle, with the welcomer opposite the caregiver to encourage less verbal group members to interact. The co-worker sits next to the person who needs constant touching in order to remain in the group. Refreshments should be placed near the group, but not so close that some group member might eat before the others.

CONDUCTING A VALIDATION GROUP MEETING

Validation groups must meet at least once each week, for at least 20 minutes. The maximum meeting time is 1 hour. Each meeting has a new life, and the length of the meeting fluctuates, depending on the energy level of group members.

Before the Group Meeting

Before each meeting, the validating caregiver should do the following:

1. Observe each group member to pick up important clues.

2. Check with staff to determine the physical and emotional condition of group members. For example, if a group member was verbally abused by another resident just before the meeting, this can be expressed and resolved with the help of other group members and can be the topic for the day.

3. Relate the topic to be discussed or problem to be solved to a specific group member. Introduce the topic by asking a verbal, nurturing group member to help the person who needs nurturing. Problem solving leads to increased feelings of independence and self-worth.

4. Use Validation Technique 1: Centering. A group leader who is tired, angry, or sad cannot take in the feelings of disoriented old-old people. The caregiver must acknowledge his or her feelings, closet them, Center, and then tune in to the feelings of each group member, as well as the feelings of the group as a whole. The caregiver must focus all of his or her energy on the disoriented old-old group members.

During the Group Meeting

Phase 1: Birth of the Group—Creating Energy (5–15 minutes)

1. The caregiver greets each person in the circle, using the person's last name (e.g., "Mrs. Jones") to give dignity, unless the person specifically asks to be called by his or her first name. The caregiver uses touch, eye contact, and reinforces each participant's role in the group. *Example:* "Hello, Mrs. Smith. I'm Naomi Feil. It's good to see you. Something wonderful must have happened. You look so happy. Will you be our welcomer? Next to you is Mr. Jones, and he's going to help us with the singing. Right, Mr. Jones?"

   The caregiver moves on to the next person. Individuals forget their roles from week to week, but once they begin to welcome, or start the song, or pass the cookies, they perform smoothly with grace. Each week, they perform roles with more assurance and spontaneity.

2. The caregiver encourages group members to hold hands throughout the meeting. This touching often stimulates eye contact and speech and strengthens relationships.

3. The caregiver helps the welcomer rise. The welcomer greets the group. Rising gives the welcomer status.

4. The caregiver asks the song leader to begin the song. The caregiver asks, "Shall we sing 'You Are My Sunshine?'" The song leader often begins the song spontaneously. If the song leader has forgotten the beginning, the caregiver focuses, with close eye contact with the song leader, and begins to sing. The song leader soon sings each word, and the caregiver continues focusing energy on the song

leader, using direct eye contact, mirroring the movement of the song leader's lower lip and the expression in his or her eyes, his or her pitch, and tempo. This establishes the song leader's role and status in the group. Group members will also follow the song leader, giving the song leader dignity and self-worth. The song leader will lead the group in three or four songs to build group energy.

5. The caregiver asks the poet or prayer leader to recite a prayer or poem.

Phase 2: Life of the Group—Verbal Interactions (5–10 minutes)

1. The caregiver introduces the topic by asking the nurturing verbal welcomer to help an individual with a universal problem, such as how to overcome loneliness. The caregiver engages as many group members as possible to help solve the problem, asking them how they combat loneliness, and how they find comfort. Each person can respond on some level, to the maximum of his or her capacity.

2. The validating caregiver summarizes the comments of the group, praising group members who have helped solve the problem.

Phase 3: Movement and Rhythms (3–20 minutes)

1. The caregiver asks the dance leader or rhythm band leader to take the instrument, or helps him or her rise to dance.

2. The co-worker and caregiver help each person rise and move in a circle, led by the dance leader.

3. The dance leader can begin throwing the bean bag or soft ball.

4. After movement, there can be finger painting, working with clay, planting, and so on.

Phase 4: Closing of the Group, with Anticipation for the Next Meeting (5–15 minutes)

1. The caregiver asks the song leader to begin the closing song.

2. The caregiver helps the host or hostess rise and pass the refreshments. This stimulates more activity, verbal interactions, eye contact, and feelings of sociability and heightened energy.

3. The caregiver helps the welcomer rise and say goodbye to the group, with warm wishes, anticipating the next meeting.

4. The song leader sings an upbeat song, during which group members hold hands.

5. The caregiver says goodbye to each member individually, touching each one and mentioning that he or she looks forward to the next meeting.

6. The nursing staff helps by transporting members back to the floor.

Coping with Problems During the Group Meeting

Very often, problems arise during a group meeting. To resolve these problems, the caregiver should:

1. Confront angry feelings openly. Sometimes, group participants are angry before the group meeting begins. Their lips will be tight, their bodies rigid, their hands held tight, their jaws thrust forward. Participants who are usually verbal will refuse to speak or will speak in a clipped manner. Often, one group member's objectionable behavior (e.g., yelling, pacing, swearing, undressing) will anger the rest of the group. The validating caregiver should confront these angry feelings directly (e.g., "Mrs. Green, you don't want to answer me. You seem angry.").

2. Match the feelings of the group by mirroring participants' movements. When a caregiver notices that a group member is uncomfortable, he or she should imitate the person's movements. When a group member makes a fist, for example, the caregiver should make a fist. This assures the group member that his or her anger is acceptable and encourages the member to share his or her feelings. By mirroring an unacceptable behavior, the caregiver makes the group member aware of what he or she is doing, as the following example shows:

   Mrs. Snow begins to take off her clothes during the group meeting. The caregiver turns to Mrs. Green, another group member and asks, "Does Mrs. Snow's unbuttoning her dress make you angry? What can we do about it? Shall we ask her what she is feeling?" She then turns to Mrs. Snow. "Mrs. Snow, you are making Mrs. Green very angry by unbuttoning your dress." The caregiver then demonstrates unbuttoning and buttoning to help Mrs. Snow become aware of her behavior. Mrs. Snow stops undressing herself as she watches the caregiver. As Mrs. Snow watches, the caregiver tries to understand the feelings underlying Mrs.

*Snow's behavior. "Do you feel all tied up?" she asks.
"Does unbuttoning your dress make you feel freer?"
Mrs. Snow nods. "Mrs. Snow feels all tied up," explains
the caregiver. "Do you ever feel tied up or closed in,
Mrs. Green?"*

The caregiver continues to explore the group members' feelings until all of the participants have vented their feelings. Having helped the group members express their feelings of anger or sadness, the caregiver can then proceed with the opening ritual.

After the Group Meeting

It is important to move members into a social situation—such as lunch, a large musical program, or a religious service—immediately after the group meeting. If members are isolated in their rooms after the meeting, they will feel abandoned and often may begin to exhibit negative behaviors. They may feel rejected after having been part of a warm, social, family group. After the group meeting, the caregiver and co-worker fill in the Validation group evaluation form, (see page 261) to prepare for the next meeting. Between meetings, the caregiver should continue individual Validation with specific treatment plans for each group member, so that nursing staff can continue the Validation on an individual basis. For example, a specific plan for Mr. Jones might read: "Touch Mr. Jones gently on the cheek, fingers rotating upward, 20 strokes. He misses his mother, and this touch will elicit eye contact. He will stop crying. Sing three songs to him: 'You Are My Sunshine,' 'Jesus Loves Me,' and 'Lullaby and Goodnight.'" This individual Validation takes no more than 3 minutes.

Dealing with Death or
the Departure of the Validation Worker

Disoriented old-old people rarely mourn when a group member dies or when the caregiver leaves. This is because they substitute one person for another, unable to distinguish relationships. When a group member dies, the caregiver meets with nursing, social service, and activities staff to find a replacement. Usually, group members will not remember the person who has left. They will accept a new group member, providing that the person is in Time Confusion and is not abusive. If a new caregiver is needed, he or she must be nurturing and respectful; group members will quickly transfer trust to the new caregiver who validates them. If the worker is not replaced, group members will quickly regress.

EXAMPLE OF A VALIDATION GROUP

(See the video *The More We Get Together*, 1980, Feil Productions.)
     The worker moves around the circle, introducing herself and saying the name of each group member. Group members take each other's hands, responding to the genuine, close eye contact, touch, and nurturing voice tone of the worker. The worker reinforces group roles. After she has greeted each group member, she turns to the Welcomer, Mrs. Flanigan.

Worker: Mrs. Flanigan, you are our Welcomer. You start us out on the right foot. Will you stand up and say a few words of welcome to make everyone feel at home?
Mrs. Flanigan: Ladies, we all have flumkin baggin's disease. That's a disease of old age. When you get old, you have good imagination and smelly piss.

Worker: *(Centering)* That's a very interesting disease, Mrs. Flanigan. How did you discover that?

Mrs. Flanigan: I just went to the bathroom, and it came to me.

Mr. Small: She's right. That old lady never smelled so bad when she was a young girl.

Worker: Is that one of the hardest things to take when you get old?

Mr. Small: I don't know, lady. I'm just telling you what I smell, that's all.

Mrs. Kappe: Well, it's better to be old, then it doesn't matter what you do!

Mrs. Falk: *(to Mrs. Kappe)* At your age, you should know better.

Mrs. Kappe: I don't know what you mean. I'm under 25.

Mrs. Falk: You should know better than to take other people's husbands. Bitch!

Mr. Small: That's a bad word, lady. Shame on you.

Mrs. Kappe: You're crazy if you're inadequate, and you're crazy if you're not, so what's the difference?

Mr. Small: I'm burning up, lady. I'm drowning.

Mrs. Smith: Oh, shut up and drop dead!

A silence falls over the group. The Validation worker rephrases and summarizes, matching the emotion of group members.

Worker: Mrs. Falk, you're angry because "she" stole your husband, and Mr. Small, you feel that people should control their emotions. Sometimes you feel as if you were dead— burning up inside? Mrs. Smith, do you ever feel as if you were dead?

Mrs. Smith: Drop dead. All of you. And shut up.

Worker: Are you angry at us all, Mrs. Smith, because we told each other how we feel?

Mrs. Smith: Yes. Behave. All of you. Nobody acts like a human being.

Mr. Small: Shut up yourself, bitch.

Mrs. Smith: Drop dead.

Worker: Mr. Small, you're angry at Mrs. Smith because she doesn't like the way we talk, is that it?

Mr. Small: That's it, lady. I can talk any way I like.

Worker: Mrs. Smith, do you think everyone has a right to talk any way they like?

Mrs. Smith: Well, if they behave themselves.

Worker: *(to the nurturing welcomer, who solves all problems for the group)* Mrs. Flanigan, can you help us? Shall we say what we think, or shall we shut up?

Mrs. Flanigan: Both. I think we should do both. And behave.

Worker: Thank you, Mrs. Flanigan. You always help us out in a tight spot. Do you think we have solved the problem? Have we talked enough?

Mr. Small: It's enough, lady. Let's sing a song, huh?

Worker: That's a great idea! You're our song leader, Mr. Small. What about "The More We Get Together?"

Mr. Small sings in a loud, joyful voice. The worker helps group members hold hands, and they sing lustily together. The group has solved a problem, and they feel close. They sing three or four songs. They have talked enough. The worker's planned topic was to talk about loneliness, but the worker abandons her plan, moving with the rhythm of the group and Mrs. Falk's need to express anger that had been bottled up for many years. Mrs. Falk's husband had hurt her by womanizing, many years ago, and Mrs. Falk now uses Mrs. Kappe in present time to vent her anger. Mrs. Falk will express her anger again and again in the group, until she feels relieved. She will not hit out, and her anger will be expressed with words, in a socially acceptable way in the Validation group. Before joining the Validation group, Mrs. Falk would swear and strike women she thought had taken away her husband.

The worker asks the dance leader to lead the group in a circle dance to the rhythm of a Mitch Miller tape. The co-worker dances with the wheelchair residents, while the worker dances with group members who can bear weight.

After three circle dances, the worker asks the hostess to serve refreshments. Mrs. Falk, a former entertainer, is the hostess. She passes out the juice and cookies with style, permitting group members to take only one cookie at a time. As she passes out the cookies, she maintains eye contact and her speech increases. She moves around the circle, relishing her role. Before becoming the hostess, Mrs. Falk would not bear weight, although she could walk. In her role as hostess, she is motivated to move, interacting with others, both in and outside the Validation group.

Before closing the meeting, the worker asks the song leader to begin singing "Daisy." The group sings three or four songs, with heightened energy and joy. Energized by the movement, the food, the conversation, and the self-respect that they feel at being heard, the group feels satisfied. The meeting is now ready to end. The worker summarizes.

Worker: This was a wonderful meeting. Mrs. Flanigan, you helped us learn that we can say what we feel and still not hurt other people. Mrs. Falk, you feel badly when another woman took your husband. Do you think we can talk about it some more next week?

Mrs. Falk: Certainly. She should know what she did.

Worker: *(using the ambiguous pronoun "she")* She hurt you very much, and you never told her, and now it's time to get it off your chest, is that right?

Mrs. Falk: You said a mouthful.

Worker: *(planning for the next meeting)* Next week, we'll talk about taking other people's husbands and what to tell people when they hurt us. Mrs. Smith, we hurt you when we used bad words, didn't we?

Mrs. Smith: *(nodding)* It's disgusting. Really disgusting.

Mr. Small: That's a good one, lady. Nobody hurts me and gets away with it.

Worker: *(to help Mrs. Kappe express her feelings)* Mrs. Kappe, when your feelings get hurt, do you tell someone how you feel?

Mrs. Kappe: I do, honey. I do. Don't worry about me.

Worker: Do you think we're ready to end our meeting?

Mr. Small: Let's end it. I'll sing another song.

Worker: What about "Let Me Call You Sweetheart?"

Mr. Small begins singing immediately, and the group joins in, holding hands and swaying to the music. The worker asks Mrs. Flanigan, the welcomer, to say a few words to close the meeting after the song has ended.

Mrs. Flanigan: Well, we've all surrounded ourselves with thoughts. When bad ones come, we spit it out and then we don't smell so bad. Goody.

The worker shakes hands with each group member, reinforcing each person's contribution, anticipating another good time next week. Nursing assistants who understand the need for the Validation group are ready to take the group members to the dining room for lunch. The nursing staff has seen the benefits of the Validation group. Mr. Small no longer yells at night. Mrs. Falk no longer hits other women.

Mrs. Smith swears less, and all group members interact more with others after the group meeting. The Validation group has lasted 45 minutes and meets each week. Members keep the same roles until they die. This Validation group has been going for the past 10 years.

WHO CAN PRACTICE VALIDATION?

Most people find that they need training in Validation to integrate the theory and techniques in practice. Certified Validation teachers offer courses in Validation. There are four levels of certification. Each level builds on the experience and knowledge gained from the preceding course. The requirements[1] follow.

Level 1: Validation Worker

- Take part in a Validation training course

- Practice individual Validation for at least 6 months

- Show documentation of practical work experience

- Pass written and practical examinations

Level 2: Validation Group Practitioner

- Show Level 1 certification or equivalent

- Take part in a group Validation training course

- Practice group Validation for at least 6 months

- Pass written and practical examinations

---

[1] For certification information, contact the Validation Training Center, George M. Leader Institute, 830 Cherry Drive, Hershey, PA 17033; telephone (717) 533-2474; or the Validation Training Center at Virginia Commonwealth University, 1101 East Marshal Street, Post Office Box 980568, Richmond, VA 23298; telephone (804) 828-5188. For workshop information, contact Naomi Feil, 21987 Byron Road East, Shaker Heights, OH 44122; telephone (216) 561-0357.

Level 3: Validation Teacher

- Show Level 2 certification
- Have some previous teaching experience
- Take part in a Validation teacher's training course
- Pass written and practical examinations
- Take part in co-training

Level 4: Validation Master

- Show Level 3 certification
- Complete at least 3 years as a Validation teacher
- Be authorized by the Validation Training Institute

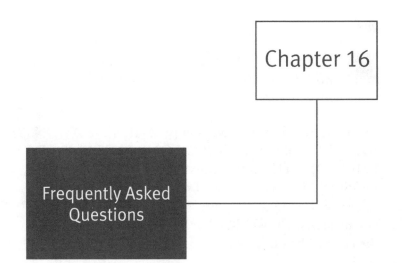

Chapter 16

Frequently Asked Questions

I've tried Validation, but my client won't talk with me. Why doesn't it work?

Which Validation techniques did you use? Did you Center and establish the Stage of Disorientation? If the old person is in Stage 2 or 3, verbal techniques may not work. If your clients feel that you are not empathetic, techniques are useless. Validation workers must enter the world of the old person, match their emotions, and then use verbal or nonverbal techniques.

■ *I feel uncomfortable when my client cries when I validate her. Isn't it bad for old people to get so worked up?*

The basic principle in Validation is: WHEN EMOTIONS ARE EXPRESSED AND SOMEONE LISTENS WITH EMPATHY, THE EMOTIONS ARE RELIEVED. THE PERSON FEELS BETTER. If you are uncomfortable with strong emotions and you wish to help your client feel better, you must first CENTER, release your own discomfort, and then feel with your client.

■ *How do I know when a disoriented old person is using a symbol?*

When an old disoriented person uses an object—a piece of clothing, a part of their body, or another person—and expresses strong emotions that are not related to present time, then the old person is using a symbol.

■ *I've been doing Validation instinctively for years. Why should I take a course to learn it?*

Validation is a theory, a method, and an attitude. You may have the validating attitude—accepting and respecting the old person where they are—however, in order to use the techniques it is vital to learn the depth of Validation theory. In a course, you learn to integrate the principles of Validation with practice. You need feedback and supervision in order to really learn the techniques.

You say, "don't ever lie," but does that mean pretending to agree with Mrs. Smith when she says, "My mother is waiting for me?" How do you reconcile these conflicting ideas?

Validation does not mean pretending or agreeing or disagreeing. When you validate someone, you listen to them, without adding your own reality. You enter into the reality of the disoriented old person. You help disoriented old people express themselves in order to work through unresolved relationships. In your example you might say, "What do you need to do for your mother?"

Our patients feel good here. Can you prove that Validation will help them feel better?

You can use the Validation group evaluation form in Chapter 15 to find out if Validation is restoring well-being. Rate the person from 0 to 4. If the old person complains less, communicates more, cries less, smiles more, and so forth after Validation, then you know that the Validation techniques are helping.

It seems like you think Validation is the only method there is. Why can't I use other methods or therapies?

You can and should. There is no single, fool-proof method for disoriented older people. Music, movement, and activities are just a few other helping methods. Maloriented old people often respond to Remotivation and Reminiscing groups. Validation is just one effective method to know to help disoriented people restore communication and maintain dignity.

■ *Is Validation a therapy or a method?*

Validation is a theory, a method, and an attitude—a theory that very old people need to resolve unfinished issues before death; a method with 15 helping techniques; and an attitude of respect for the disoriented old person. Validation does not give the old person insight or try to cure him or her, as in psychotherapy. However, Validation is therapeutic in that it lessens agitation, restores well-being, and maintains communication.

■ *How do I know if I'm doing it right?*

If your client feels better, is less agitated, complains less, communicates more, and relates to others positively, then you are doing Validation correctly.

■ *How do I handle someone who is acting aggressively?*

First, you Center yourself, to rid yourself of your own emotions. Then, if the person is verbal, you Rephrase while matching the emotion in your voice tone and your body. Use Mirroring if the person is nonverbal. It is important that you not try to calm the person. Everyone has a right to be angry.

Mr. Tinker doesn't speak at all. How can I understand him?

First, Center, to clear away your own preconceptions. Then, look at Mr. Tinker from top to toe. What is he feeling? You can often tell what is going on inside a person by a careful observation of his or her physical characteristics, this is called a *calibration.* For example: Are his lips pursed? Quivering? Set in a straight line? If they are set in a straight line, he may be angry. Say his emotion out loud, *with* emotion. "You are so angry? Did someone hurt you?" If you feel Mr. Tinker's anger, he will know it. He knows that you are on his wavelength. He will open his eyes and look at you. This is the beginning of communication.

What is the difference between an hallucination and the use of the eidetic image by disoriented old-old people?

An eidetic image is a visual image retained in the memory. The image is a projection of old memories and is based on the personal history of the individual, usually connected to some unfinished issues from the past. A hallucination does not necessarily have to do with the past or personal history of the individual. Validation theory states that disoriented old-old people stimulate eidetic images in order to resolve unfinished issues, thus making this a healthy process.

Experiences of
Professionals in the
United States and
Abroad

IMPLEMENTING VALIDATION AT COUNTRY MEADOWS RETIREMENT COMMUNITIES

*Rita Altman R.N., C.G.P., Corporate Director of Country Meadows
(Dementia Care Programs)*

Country Meadows Retirement Communities, founded in 1983, is owned and operated by the family of former Pennsylvania Governor George M. Leader. We have 3,000 residents at 33 facilities throughout Pennsylvania and will open a campus in Frederick, Maryland, in April, 2002. Country Meadows has been actively using the Validation method since 1999.

In 1998, Naomi Feil was invited to Country Meadows to present her second series of 2-day Validation seminars at each of our 10 campuses. I had the privilege of meeting Naomi at the airport, and on the way to her hotel we stopped at one of our facilities for a brief tour. We visited a Meadows Living Center where all of the residents had some degree of dementia. In less than 1 hour of observing Naomi, I was convinced that Validation was the best method of communication that I had ever seen with this population of residents. Undoubtedly, I was most impressed with the way that Naomi totally immersed herself in conversation with every person that she spoke with, giving each one her total, undivided attention. I believe that each resident knew that someone was genuinely listening to him or her and validating his or her feelings.

Now that I understand Validation, I realize that Naomi was truly Centered as she spoke with each person. Her eyes were wide open and completely focused on each individual, and she seemed to be mirroring the expression on his or her face. Within moments of being Validated by Naomi, each person responded by making better eye contact and standing or sitting more erectly. They experienced being truly acknowledged and valued, which made them appear more self-confident and maintain more dignity. Having observed this, I can recall thinking that I wanted all of our caregivers to be trained in this method of communication because all of our residents deserved to be heard and responded to by caregivers who knew Validation.

Michael Leader, the president and chief executive officer of Country Meadows, believed so strongly in this empathetic form of communication that in 1999 he decided that we should become an authorized Validation Training Organization with the goal of advancing Validation. In fact, since 1999, several of our co-workers and others from all over the country have attended the Validation training sessions that are conducted at Country Meadows and taught by Naomi Feil and Vicki de Klerk-Rubin. As a result, several Country Meadows co-workers are now certified Validation workers and certified group practitioners. They provide individual and group Validation at many of our facilities where other co-workers are now learning about Validation by their example.

Validation principles are also interwoven throughout all of the modules of our company's dementia care training, which every new co-worker receives within their first 90 days of employment. In addition, we provide ongoing quarterly training programs that also contain Validation principles and techniques. In 2002, we will introduce a basic Validation training module at each of our facilities on a quarterly basis. One of our co-workers, Deb Kunkel, C.V.W., has already developed and piloted this four-part series at our Leader Heights campus.

One of the most requested training sessions is on difficult behaviors. We have developed a Validation approach to difficult behaviors in which our caregivers are trained to link the behavior with the resident's unmet need. Our co-workers are challenged to enter the world of the resident and to mirror his or her feelings. Instead of diversion and redirection or therapeutic lies, our caregivers are taught that every elderly disoriented person has wisdom and that deep inside they know the truth. We emphasize the importance of establishing trust with each resident. Family members have also been included in this process because they struggle to try to make their loved one remember by using reality with them, which only results in more frustration.

At the most basic level, we are trying to instill the attitude of empathy and the desire to establish a trusting relationship with each resident in each of our caregivers. The paradigm shift from diversion, therapeutic lying, and reality to Validation does not occur overnight. Validation is much more than principles or communication techniques, it is a philosophy of care that requires time to learn and use. However, the benefits to the residents and caregivers are immeasurable. Our co-workers have reported that using Validation has reduced resident agitation and aggression on many occasions. Validation has also resulted in the use of fewer psychotropic medications. Family members have commented that since their loved ones have been in weekly Validation group sessions, they look happier and are able to better communicate with them. When one family member observed her loved one in a Validation group, she commented that she wished that everyone in the family could see how much she was still able to contribute to the group and that she still had so much wisdom.

Country Meadows plans on conducting research to prove that Validation is beneficial, and the staff hopes that more people will use this method. Although the paradigm shift is slow in occurring, it is nonetheless occurring one Validation moment at a time.

John C. Colletti, Psy.D., President, Chapman Senior Care

The Masonic Home of Virginia is home to an ongoing Validation group culled from individuals originally referred as part of a consulting psychology service. This article describes the stages that took place in establishing the group, as well as the logistical and financial obstacles that need to be addressed by a Validation worker who is not employed by a long-term care facility.

When I began practicing as a consulting psychologist at several long-term care facilities, I was in a bind when asked to assist in treating residents who were not deemed appropriate for traditional psychotherapy (e.g., those diagnosed with Alzheimer's-type dementia as well as depressive, anxious, or behavioral disturbances). I could not, in good conscience, simply ask the treatment team to utilize medication without a behavioral intervention and, similarly, could not advocate for traditional behavior management techniques. Behavior therapy requires all shifts to observe the behavioral program's tenets (a true challenge with the current rate of staff turnover). Also, traditional behavior programs place the resident in the role of having "maladaptive" behaviors rather than simply expressing an appropriate response to the "transfer trauma" many of these residents experience. Finally, because I was not an employee of any facility, I needed to provide a treatment for which there was no payment (i.e., commercial insurance or Medicare/Medicaid do not reimburse for behavior treatment with people diagnosed with Alzheimer's-type dementia).

My search for a workable, caregiver-friendly approach to treating this population led me to read the first edition of *The Validation Breakthrough*. I immediately realized the potential of instituting this practice as it gave me hope and practical advice for the residents, staff, and families with whom I worked. After pursuing certification as a Validation worker, I began instituting short in-service training programs in the facilities that our practice served in order to begin the process of "weaning" the facility staff off of the concept of reality orientation. Meanwhile, I enrolled in the Level 2 group practitioner training course in Hershey, Pennsylvania, in the fall of 2000.

The first validation group in Virginia was started in September, 2000, at the Masonic Home of Virginia in Richmond. This nonprofit continuing care retirement community campus began in 1890 as a children's home and was converted to a home for the elderly in 1955. In May, 2001, there were 259 residents, 58 of them in the Health Care Center, a wing designated for individuals diagnosed with Alzheimer's-type dementia. Prior to Chapman Senior Care's involvement with the facility in 2000, a geriatric psychiatrist served as the consultant to the residents. When our team of psychologists began work with the facility, the social services staff immediately resonated with the idea of Validation and, as a result, arranged a series of in-service training sessions for the general staff. This cohesion with the facility staff was instrumental in ensuring an ongoing program. I presented the concept of Validation, showed the videos *Communicating with the Alzheimer's-type Population: The Validation Method* and *Myrna—The Maloriented,* (available through Health Professions Press) and disseminated a synopsis of some basic techniques prepared by an intern from Virginia Commonwealth University (VCU). From those in-services, a core group of four staff from the social services and activity departments (as well as the two interns I was working with at that time) volunteered to be part of the Validation team at the facility. I also did some training with our psychologist who gave me a list of individuals who were originally referred for a psychological evaluation but whose behaviors seemed to reflect problems with Resolution rather than mental illness.

After interviewing residents on the list with members of the Validation team and doing some more intensive training concerning the group methodology, we decided on a core group of eight residents and began to hold weekly group meetings (approximately 1 hour in length with 30 minutes debriefing with the Validation team) in a secluded parlor. Each of these residents was found to have significant dementia symptoms (consistent with Phases 2 and 3 of Resolution) as was indicated on the Mattis Dementia Rating Scale (DRS). A study is underway to measure the progress of members of the group by comparing their DRS pre- and postscores as well as their weekly progress forms.

During staff training, it was emphasized that Validation is not a "curative" model, and the benefits of Validation should not be measured in terms of "decreased maladaptive behaviors" as is prescribed with traditional behavior therapy. However, the following were seen as qualitative improvements in the residents who were treated: less need for psychotropic medication, fewer symptoms of anxiety/depression/behavioral outbursts, and increased social activity. Similarly, the staff reported more cohesion with fellow staff members and increased self-fulfillment and satisfaction with their role in the facility. Families were invited to sit in on the sessions and reported increased understanding of their loved ones due to the training they received and the effectiveness of the group intervention they saw. The group continues to meet weekly and to admit new members, and the Validation team continues to meet and grow with the support of both facility departments.

Although lack of funding continues to be a serious problem, the ability to effectively create a program to help underserved residents has helped Chapman Senior Care to grow into a large, effective practice. The volume of referrals to a practice that utilizes Validation has allowed me the ability to spend much of my time instituting Validation programs in these facilities, as well as setting up an Authorized Validation Organization through VCU's Virginia Geriatric Education Center. The future of Validation therapy in Virginia is a bright one as other facilities are now learning that the ongoing Validation program at the Masonic Home of Virginia and the ability to train new Validation workers and trainers at VCU's Virginia Geriatric Education Center has provided the promise of giving quality and caring services to a large number of individuals.

Using Validation in a 60-Bed Skilled Medicare
Facility in the Kansas City Metropolitan Area:
An Administrator's Perspective

Scott Averill, B.S., J.D., N.H.A., Administrator,
Colonial Manor of Lansing/Beverly Enterprises

Colonial Manor, a Lansing/Beverly Enterprises facility outside of Kansas City, began using Validation after its activity director introduced the administrator to the idea. The facility eventually began three Validation groups—including one led by a long-time volunteer—and holding weekly Validation team meetings.

Josephine became a resident of Colonial Manor the same day I became the Administrator—December 21, 1990. She was 86, and for some reason she immediately took a liking to a wingback chair located just outside my office. When I tried talking to her, she politely informed me that she lived at 9th Avenue and Spruce and her father was coming by to pick her up. Without giving my response a second thought, I said, "Josephine, you live at Colonial Manor now, and your father is dead," whereupon she gave me a very indignant look, pumped her arms up and down, and became visibly angry. Although I didn't know it at the time, my initial responses to Josephine (telling her she no longer lived at 9th Avenue and Spruce and that her father had died) represented a form of reality orientation. And for whatever reason, that is what was natural for me to say at the time. To say anything else would have been lying.

Such incidents went on for about 6 months until the day my activity director, Jennifer Carpenter, returned from a workshop on Validation. After just one conversation with Jennifer and skimming through Naomi Feil's book, *Validation: The Feil Method*, my approach to working with Josephine and residents like her was forever changed.

My staff and I were so enthralled by Naomi's book and what my activity director kept sharing with us that we decided to invite Naomi to our area to lead a workshop. On very short notice, we had more than 100 people registered. And what was really amazing is that unlike most continuing education seminars, where participants can't wait to get out of the room at the end of the day, the people in Naomi's workshop didn't want to go home when it ended. They stayed around to talk with one another and waited in line to buy Naomi's book or ask her questions.

One of the participants in that first workshop was Velma Bass, a woman who had been volunteering at Colonial Manor for more than 15 years. What she heard Naomi say that day really fit with her experience of being with many residents at Colonial Manor over the years. Within a couple of weeks, she was leading the first ever Validation group at my facility. About 3 months later, one of our Certified Nurse Aides, Lowell Dodson, had started a second group. About 5 months later, my activity director and I started co-leading a third group.

Each of our Validation groups met in a multipurpose conference room. Each meeting usually took 40–60 minutes, and we usually had five to eight residents each time. In the first several months, each group had its own members and very rarely would members of one group visit another group. Later, this changed, and several residents attended two and sometimes all three Validation groups every week. Documentation was kept for each group meeting on each individual resident. When we began our third group, we began having weekly Validation team meetings at 9:00 A.M. every Friday morning. Validation group leaders and the registered nurse who led our care plan team attended these meetings.

After Validation had been actively practiced in my facility for 18 months, I saw several areas of our operation that had been significantly affected:

1. Staff turnover had fallen markedly. Prior to introducing Validation, our annual turnover was 170%. It decreased more than 80% the first year we began Validation and remained at the lower level in the second year.

2. Staff morale, attendance, and productivity improved: No call/no shows and weekend call-ins became rare. The hassle and frustration of working with residents with dementia became less aggravating when staff members had a new way of approaching and interacting with them.

3. Family members discovered a new way of being with their loved ones that allowed them to continue to express and experience their love for one another. Validation also decreased the friction among family members that is often present when a loved one has dementia.

Within 18 months of using Validation in my facility, including the three weekly Validation group meetings, and the Validation team meeting every Friday, we knew we had barely scratched the surface—which proved to be very exciting. One of the great aspects of Validation is that it can be practiced by anyone on the staff—housekeeping, laundry, maintenance, dietary, and nursing. Our first group leader was a long-time volunteer.

Every nursing home in the United States has a federally legislated mandate to provide an environment in which each resident functions at his or her "highest practicable level." To achieve this goal is a daily challenge within all nursing homes. The ongoing practice of Validation is one of the best approaches I've found to meet this challenge.

Sheldon Pinsky, Ph.D., Chartered Psychologist, Licensed Independent Clinical Social Worker, Licensed Marriage and Family Therapist, AAMFT Clinical Member Alzheimer's & Dementia Unit

In the early 1990s, the Minnesota Veterans' Home was a nonprofit facility in Minneapolis, Minnesota, that was home to 422 male residents who had been diagnosed with Alzheimer's dementia. These residents were in the Alzheimer's and Dementia Unit, which was a separate, locked, secured unit. Some of these residents that were transferred to the Veterans' Home from private nursing homes were unable to manage their wandering, agitation, and aggressiveness. Others were transferred from Veterans Administration hospitals, other state facilities, and their own homes. Using Validation, the Veterans' Home restored dignity and a sense of self-worth to their residents.

Our approach to care was to use a multidisciplinary team that used Validation to establish empathy and rapport with our residents. This process allowed these residents to adapt comfortably to the home and taught the team to accept our residents' behaviors in order to uncover the reasons behind their emotions.

When a new resident entered the facility, I met with him and his family to assess their needs in relation to total care and care planning. As the head of the Validation team at the Veterans' Home, I then met with the Alzheimer's multidisciplinary team, which consisted of nursing, social services, dietary, medical, psychiatry, psychology, recreational, and occupational therapy staff, to formulate care plans that involved careful listening, eye contact, touch, trust, and empathy. These care plans addressed the resident's feelings and needs. I helped the team formulate treatment recommendations with specific goals and daily objectives, weekly progress summaries, and program care plans. These plans reflected the principles of Validation, as well as described the techniques, both of which are instrumental in improving the quality of life for each resident.

We used Validation both in groups and on an individual basis. Sometimes groups were preferred for Time Confused residents, whereas individual therapy was used for Maloriented, combative, and more thoroughly confused residents. Validation was very helpful in restoring our residents' dignity and in teaching our staff to understand our residents' reasons for behavior. Residents became less combative, less antisocial, and more cooperative with staff. They were no longer dangerous to themselves or others and participated in and enjoyed recreational activities that utilized the Validation approach.

In 1991, I measured the effect of Validation on the following observable behaviors: 1) yelling, 2) combativeness with other residents, 3) combativeness with staff, 4) agitation, 5) restlessness, 6) delusions, 7) paranoia, 8) repetitive physical movements (e.g., wandering, picking up imaginary objects), 9) depression, and 10) anxiety. Residents who were Validated for 4 weeks showed a decrease in these behaviors and were more communicative, less confused, and more oriented than they were before receiving Validation therapy. In contrast, residents who received reality orientation for 4 weeks showed an increase in these behaviors and were less communicative, more confused, and less oriented following therapy.

I met weekly with family members, the resident psychiatrist, the doctor, nurses, and social workers to review the progress of each resident and to determine how to decrease their maladaptive behavior. I encouraged all families to visit the home at least three times a week during lunch, dinner, or recreational programs so that they could observe how each resident was responding to Validation. My goal was to give each resident and family member a renewed sense of self-worth and to establish communication between residents and families so they could share their feelings and understand their roles in the relationship.

Validation makes it possible for both residents and their families to cope with disorientation. Family members have told me that, following Validation, they are better able to tolerate the "living death" label given to those with Alzheimer's dementia because they see in themselves and in their disoriented relatives a sense of connecting with the past, present, and future.

Mary Bayer RN-C, Co-owner of the Sandy River Alliance Nursing Care Centers; Karen Leary, LSW; Tina Mikkelsen, CTR.S.; Meg Nobel, R.N.; and Cheryl Martin, Recreational Therapist, Woodford Park Nursing Care Center in Portland, Maine

Woodford Park Nursing Care Center was a 154-bed proprietary nursing home located in an established residential neighborhood in Portland, Maine when it was purchased by Sandy River Alliance Nursing Care Centers in 1989. At the time of the purchase, the facility was experiencing severe staffing problems, the quality of the food was poor, the housekeeping barely met minimum standards, and the physical environment was dark and dingy. Since appropriate gatekeeping had not been practiced in the screening of potential admissions, at least 75% of the residents required a heavy level of care. Throughout the facility, residents were housed randomly, with little thought given to diagnosis or nursing care needs. Many of the residents with dementia appeared extremely disoriented, noisy, frightened, and demanding of other residents, families, and staff. To deal with the unusually large number of disoriented residents, staff used reality orientation, something the new owners sought to change upon taking over.

Before new owners took over Woodford Park, reality orientation had been used with all residents, whether they were disoriented or not. The new owners found reality orientation to be of little benefit, since the oriented residents were already aware of what was being discussed and the disoriented residents seemed to pay little, if any, attention to the person conducting the group. Staff failed to listen to residents, but instead tried to convince confused residents that their fears or wishes were not real. The result was agitation, arguing, and outbursts from the residents and increased frustration and burnout on the part of the staff.

The new owners were familiar with the work of Naomi Feil and decided to institute Validation at Woodford Park, since they had had good results with the approach at another home they owned. One Validation group was started by staff familiar with Validation, and a 2-day Validation workshop was held for the administrators, nursing administrators, social workers, and recreational therapy staff in all of the nursing homes owned by Sandy River. Naomi Feil was invited to come as teacher and consultant.

The staff of Woodford Park came back from the workshop with lots of ideas and enthusiasm. All were busy with their jobs, however, and it was not clear how their excitement could be turned into a program. Fortunately, the facility's administrator took the lead, calling together all of the staff who had attended the workshop and establishing a Validation team. This team consisted of a licensed social worker, a nurse, and a recreational therapist.

The team agreed that the first goal was to assess every resident in the facility who had a documented state of confusion. Using the facility's computerized care plans, the team easily identified those residents who were potential Validation candidates. So that the interdisciplinary teams would not be overwhelmed, each team was asked to assess one resident for Validation. The needs of each resident would then be addressed in the plan of care and recorded on the Kardex. The resident would also be assessed for appropriateness in a Validation group, and the resident's name and a copy of the group assessment would be submitted to the Validation team.

A "Song of the Week" was selected and photocopies were distributed on the units so that all staff could learn era-appropriate songs to sing with residents. The words were posted on each unit and nursing assistants were encouraged to sing along with residents as they waited together in the dining rooms before meals. Initially, some of the nursing assistants were a bit shy, but most joined in and appeared to enjoy the experience of seeing the residents perk up and sing old, familiar tunes.

The team also decided to show videotapes about Validation to as many staff as possible. This was done by holding a month-long "Validation Film Festival." Fliers were posted around the facility and sent to families of residents. Each week, one of the team members showed a different videotape on Validation and lead a discussion with the viewers. On the evening and night shifts, the nursing supervisors showed the videotapes. In this way, all interested staff and families were included in the viewing of the Validation videotapes.

A brief in-service was held on one of the heaviest care units during a staff meeting. Because so many staff members were convinced that reality orientation was the "way to go" with disoriented residents, the Validation team decided to perform a role-play that would highlight the difference between reality orientation and Validation. The recreational therapist on our team played the confused resident and the social worker demonstrated an intervention using reality orientation. The two ended up in a power struggle with the usual outcome—anger and frustration for both. The two then replayed the same scene using Validation as the means of communication in order to demonstrate the superior effectiveness of Validation. This brief meeting inspired curiosity from other staff, which encouraged us to hold a 1-hour in-service for all interested staff.

As a result of Validation, we grew to have had fewer behavioral problems with our disoriented residents and were able to decrease the use of physical and chemical restraints. Notes kept during the first year reveal the results of our groups:

> For the past year, our Validation group, the "group of love," has been meeting every Thursday for 30–45 minutes. Friendships have developed, and the residents are affectionate and helpful with each other. The subject of love and the importance of being loved comes up frequently. This is how our name for the group evolved.
>
> Love and friendship are discussed frequently and the participants talk a lot about childhood memories, husbands, loneliness, death, and family relationships. Handholding appears to bring them closer to each other and make them feel more comfortable.
>
> Because of the dynamics of the group, "normal" conversations hardly ever occur. Group leaders are constantly trying to make sense of words they don't understand. This sometimes leads us astray of the topic, but the group leader usually tries to bring us back to the topic, so that new ideas and memories can be stimulated.
>
> We try to give everyone in the group a role. These roles include the poet, the song leader, the chairperson, the napkin passer, and the snack passer.
>
> We have had much success with music and songs, particularly songs that trigger memories of the past. Everyone in our group enjoys singing. Even if they don't know the words they hum along or tap their hands and feet.
>
> Visual objects have also been successful: flowers, pictures, musical instruments, or any objects that can be passed around to one another. We often pass a sponge ball around and the group members have fun laughing, pretending they are going to throw a ball to one person and then throwing it to another. This brings some humor to our group.

> *The snack at the end of the group is also a time for sharing. One resident has the role of passing out napkins, and another has the role of passing out the snacks. Leaders help pour the juice.*
>
> *We have had some problems with our group. Often, group members don't show up to the meetings. Most of the time, this is because they are too sick to attend. When one member is missing, it is noticed by the other members and morale is low.*
>
> *Another problem is the residents who are hard of hearing and "patter talk." They don't seem to know what's being said unless we repeat it to them. Conversation can't flow, and we sometimes need to rearrange seating.*
>
> *Overall, though, our group has been a big success, and our residents look forward to its meeting.*

Aside from the cost of the workshops and the purchase of the Validation videotapes, the cost of initiating this program in our facility was minimal. The time and effort spent in providing continuing in-service education regarding Validation was time that we would have had to spend solving the many difficulties encountered if techniques other than Validation had been used with our disoriented residents.

In this facility, both staff and families discovered that there really is a communication approach that works with disoriented elderly people. Although we may not have been able to decrease the confusion of every resident in our facility, our staff knew that they could help each resident at least "hold the line." Because of Validation, our residents did not have to fear becoming the "living dead" people seen in nursing homes around the world.

Stephen Snow, Ph.D., R.D.T., Drama Therapist

The Wartburg Lutheran Home for the Aging, a nonprofit nursing home located in Brooklyn, New York, had been serving elderly people since 1875. In the 1980s, Wartburg, was a gardened oasis in the middle of a tough urban neighborhood and was home to 225 residents. About a third of these residents had some kind of dementia, and all were integrated into the general population of the home. In 1989, a drama therapist on the staff, attracted to Validation because of its use of role playing, started the first Validation group. Several groups, including one conducted in Spanish, were eventually developed.

Validation was introduced at Wartburg after I saw a videotape by Naomi Feil. At the time, I was completing my doctorate at New York University and was working at Wartburg as a drama therapist. I immediately recognized the connections between Validation and drama therapy. Validation was drama therapy in action!

In 1989, in collaboration with my colleague, Raymond Johnson, M.S.W., I initiated our first Validation group. Six disoriented old-old residents participated and almost immediately enjoyed and developed the roles they were assigned. It was magical to watch a disoriented 90-year-old man with a "gift for gab" deliver a well-received opening speech as the "chairperson" of the group; to observe a severely demented 90-year-old woman, who had been a singer in her 20s, come to life as the "song leader." All of the group members responded positively to the peer support approach and to the highly structured ritual of the Validation group.

I led these groups with Ray Johnson. During the weekly group meeting we alternated roles, as one of us led the group while the other took notes on the effectiveness of the techniques, the group dynamics, and the response of the residents. We found this weekly alternating of positions to be very helpful as it allowed each of us to critique the other as group leader. We augmented our knowledge of Validation by viewing the videotapes, reviewing the literature, and attending Validation workshops.

The administration at Wartburg was very supportive of our efforts. In the spring of 1990, a small grant was secured that made it possible to bring Naomi Feil to the facility. Her all-day workshop generated tremendous enthusiasm in the staff and could have served as a catalyst for the expansion of the program throughout the facility had we taken more initiative.

Perhaps the best way to reveal how effective Validation was at Wartburg is to relate an incident from one of our group meetings:

> *In the middle of one session, a 90-year-old Time Confused woman began to weep uncontrollably. Her son was at home, she said, there was no food in the house, she had no money, and she wanted to kill herself. She was distraught and clearly experiencing painful emotions. In fact, she was reliving a traumatic experience that had occurred 50 years earlier! I will never forget the way her group peers tried to console her. The "nurturing mother" in the group gently reached out to comfort her. The "chairperson" consolidated the efforts of all of the group members to help her resolve the problem. The genuine respect she received from all present enabled her to gain a new sense of peace and self-confidence. The tears went away, her*

feelings were validated, and she was able to let go of the past.

By 1990, we had expanded the program to three weekly groups, one of which was developed for the Spanish-speaking residents at Wartburg and was conducted completely in Spanish. By 1991, we had five regular weekly groups running and the program continued to benefit both staff and residents at Wartburg.

Rose Boron, LPN, CVT, Rural Outreach Coordinator,
Wisconsin Alzheimer's Information & Training Center

In the early 1990s, Heritage Haven Care Center was a 155-bed, for-profit long-term care facility in rural Wisconsin. Of its 66 residents with dementia, 28 resided in a special care unit and 38 were mainstreamed with other residents.

For many years, staff at Heritage Haven used reality orientation with our disoriented residents. Encountering a resident who refused to be fed and instead fed her doll, staff would try to convince the resident that she really didn't need to feed her doll: "Mrs. Johnson, I know that you like to carry your doll around and pretend that it is your daughter, but it's time for lunch now. Your daughter is a grown woman with children of her own. So let's put the doll on your bed for now and you can play with it after you eat a nice lunch."

Although the intent would have been to orient the resident to reality, the effect of such an approach was to strip the resident of what may have been her most important role in life, motherhood. This approach not only failed to orient the resident to reality but also robbed the resident of the only comfort she had. Disoriented residents like Mrs. Johnson often choose to re-enact a time in their life when they were needed, when they were the best at something, when they had worth. These memories are intact and are more acceptable and more pleasant than the present.

After many unsatisfactory experiences with reality orientation, the staff at Heritage Haven recognized that they seemed to be concentrating on the residents' losses and

319

weaknesses rather than on their remaining skills. By using reality orientation, the staff only reminded Mrs. Johnson that she no longer had a small baby and that no one depended on her. We reminded her that she was dependent on us.

Our staff also noticed that families seemed to become particularly frustrated by the failure of reality orientation to benefit their relatives with dementia. Many families refuse to accept dementia and are aggressive in using reality orientation. These families deny the fact that their relatives no longer perceive the same reality they do and become frustrated when they can not "bring Mom to her senses."

We sought something better for our residents and turned to Validation. We sought an approach that would allow our residents to retain their self-esteem and that would help them find a reason to continue living. We sought a way of preventing our residents from withdrawing further into themselves and deteriorating into Vegetation.

To implement Validation at Heritage Haven, we invited all interested staff, families, and volunteers to attend a workshop in which the concept of Validation was introduced. The role of the Validation team was explained, and staff who were interested in being trained in Validation were asked to contact me. The 15 staff members who expressed interest in Validation included the activities director, a nurse, several nursing assistants, and staff from the dietary, laundry, maintenance, activities, and social service departments. All attended an 8-hour training program, held 2 hours each week for 4 weeks.

Having trained our team, we then looked for residents who we thought would benefit from Validation. The cognitive levels of prospective participants were assessed during interviews with the group leader and all of the prospective participants were observed by the entire team. Careful selection and matching of participants allowed residents at each level of Resolution to play an active role in the Validation group we established. Our purpose in forming this group was to provide a setting in which residents, who may not have felt comfortable interacting socially in the larger nursing home setting, would be able to socialize. The goal was to meet the individual needs of each resident.

Prior to holding our first meeting, goals for each resident were established by the Validation team. These goals became part of the resident's clinical record.

The Validation group met weekly in a conference room on the dementia unit. These meetings lasted 40 minutes. Validation techniques were used to provide opportunities to reminisce, to talk, and to share common feelings that emphasized the residents' strengths and needs. Weekly progress notes of these meetings were kept by the Validation team. For individual residents, the team documented what types of behaviors the resident engaged in when upset, what external stimuli seemed to cause the behavior to occur, what Validation techniques were used, and the effects of these techniques.

After several months of Validation, we observed several notable changes:

- Our residents regained their dignity and were able to control their behavior.

- The number of explosive behavioral responses decreased, and we were able to use fewer physical restraints and psychotropic medications.

- Staff found it easier to work with residents with dementia and experienced less burnout.

- Staff learned to identify residents' attempts to "tie up" life issues and prepare for death and learned to use Validation to help residents do so.

- Staff morale rose.

- Staff productivity rose.

- Staff turnover fell.

- Staff became aware of their own aging and learned to prepare for their own old age.

- Families of residents gained empathy for their loved ones and learned to cope with their own losses and to assist their family members in resolving past conflicts.

- Families learned to use Validation techniques to help prevent their loved ones from withdrawing into Vegetation.

As a result of the decreased need to medicate our residents, we experienced fewer incidents of falls, decreased wandering, and decreased drug side effects. Most importantly, our residents deteriorated at a slower pace and had a higher quality of life, our staff were more satisfied with their jobs, and our families had a greater appreciation of their loved ones.

Joy Goodwin, Coordinator of Social Services and Educational Ministries, The Baptist Home, Ironton, Missouri

The Baptist Home, a nonprofit, long-term care facility in the Arcadia Valley of Missouri, was home to approximately 200 residents. It had been established in 1913. The home received no funding from the government and operated entirely out of gifts from individuals and the Missouri Baptist Convention, and from the liquidation of residents' assets. Beginning in 1980, it had used Validation to help residents cope with stress and become more oriented.

In my experience, Validation explains many of the reasons for disorientation in aging. Many people do not understand that we are dealing with the problem of *disorientation,* not *disoriented residents.* Validation was significant to us because it helped us stop trying to deal with disoriented residents, which was a very slow and often frustrating process, and start dealing with disorientation.

One of the components of disorientation in normal aging is stress, and many adults never learn to cope well with stress. Two of the greatest stresses older adults face are relocation and dramatic changes in health. During these times of extreme stress, we have applied the techniques of Validation as often as possible, *before* the individual becomes disoriented. This intervention has prevented, slowed, or reversed disorientation in the older adults in our facility.

Although Feil's target group for Validation is the disoriented population, our effort was directed toward individuals who were experiencing the most stress, whether or not they were disoriented. By using Validation at these times, we believe we prevented our residents from becoming disoriented. Rather than comparing two groups of older adults—one using Validation, the other group not using Validation—to measure the effectiveness of these techniques, we have compared our residents' status in the early 1990s with where we had been before we started using Validation. By providing support/Validation at times of stress, our program of affirmation or "mental wellness" made a difference that is measurable.

The results of Validation were dramatic in our facility. Our staff were encouraged to 1) ask questions rather than make assumptions; 2) engage in active listening; 3) believe in the potential of older adults; and 4) develop honest, open, caring relationships with our residents. We found that if the residents knew that they could depend on at least one person to accept them and validate their feelings, they felt safe enough to risk living in reality. Fewer of our residents seemed to pass into Stage 2 (Time Confusion), and many residents who had previously exhibited poor coping skills remained oriented through very stressful losses. After instituting Validation, our residents lived longer and experienced shorter periods of morbidity before death. Moreover, the overall population of our facility functioned better both physically and mentally.

Although the main focus and the most dramatic improvement from the implementation of Validation was in the area of prevention of disorientation, The Baptist Home also ran a Validation group, which began in 1982. A decade later, there was still a group for those who were disoriented enough to benefit from this type of group, although it had become more difficult to maintain a Validation group when the level of orientation had improved among the overall population.

Our experience showed that older adults living in a facility have great potential to function psychosocially, even when their bodies no longer serve them well. Caregivers who are willing to respect the autonomy of residents will find Validation an effective way of improving the morale of their staff and the quality of life of their residents.

USING VALIDATION AT ELDERCARE IN SOUTH AUSTRALIA

Alan Johns, Regional Director Eldercare, Inc., Black Forest, South Australia, and Ann Gurnett, Certified Validation Therapist, Allambi Nursing Home, South Australia

Validation was introduced in Australia in the 1980s. Since that time, it has been widely adopted in long-term care facilities, a Validation Therapy Resource and Training Centre has been established, and support groups have been created. Validation was introduced in Australia primarily through the work of two nursing consultants. A Validation Resource Centre was established in Adelaide and support groups were created in Melbourne under the auspices of the Community Aged Care Resources Centre.

There are no precise statistics on the number of organizations or individuals using Validation in Australia. In the early 1990s, it was estimated that approximately 100 organizations and 500 individuals were using Validation as part of their strategy in coping with the confused older person in a nursing home or hostel setting.

There had been very little attempt to get practitioners together who were using Validation in their workplace. One institution, however, that set up evaluation procedures was The Allambi Nursing Home in South Australia, part of the Eldercare Aged Care Facilities. Throughout the 1970s and 1980s, the dementia therapy program at Allambi was based on a philosophy of providing the optimum quality of life, maintaining the residents' cognitive skills for as long as possible, meeting the residents' psychosocial needs within a secure environment, and treating all residents with dignity and respect. The early dementia programs had been lacking in concept of self. Because of the emphasis on the group, the individual was in danger of becoming devalued, depersonalized, and isolated. Mistrustful of people surrounding them, residents were trapped in confusion of self, surroundings, and family. There were no criteria for understanding behavioral problems, such as perpetual fatigue, irritability, fear, agitation, hostility, anger, rage, and physical aggression.

Validation facilitated a clearer understanding of the meaning of these emotional exchanges, turning rigidity and cold passivity into fluid, warm activity and involvement.

The Validation program at Eldercare began at Allambi in May, 1991. It began with one-to-one therapy practices. Staff were encouraged when they saw how Validation reduced frustration, anxieties, and anger among residents and decreased pressures on staff. Other important factors noticed were improved behaviors, reduced aggression, increased interaction among residents, increased feelings of harmony, reduced stress, and heightened respect between the residents and the staff.

The first Validation group meeting was held in August 1991. It was started with eight members, a validating caregiver, and a co-worker (who was able to play the piano). The group met every Wednesday morning between 10:30 and 11:30 A.M. in a very pleasant and private room. It had been necessary to emphasize to staff the reason for the privacy, without which the group would not have been as successful. The residents remained seated at the conclusion and chattered away with increased energy while returning to their units with positive statements of enjoyment and self assurance. A close, cohesive group was maintained.

After using Validation, staff have gained clearer insight into the causes and effects of dementia and came to understand that each person is a complex combination of traits and problems. If residents accept and respond to Validation, it helps release the burden they are experiencing and assists in moving from suffering to resolution. The problems of working with residents with dementia no longer were so large that they seemed overwhelming for staff. All surrounding personnel were an integral connected part in the process with therapists, nursing staff, caregivers, relatives, volunteers, and the community.

The key requirement in funding the program was staffing costs. Other costs for the Validation group were minimal and consisted of refreshments and other miscellaneous items.

Validation Therapy was accepted in Australia with enthusiasm. The establishment of the Validation Therapy Resource and Training Centre in Adelaide provides a reliable base for both workers in the long-term care field and family caregivers to obtain information on Validation via videos and books. The establishment of support groups in 1992 through the Community Aged Care Resources Centre in Victoria assisted workers in sharing knowledge and issues of Validation Therapy. The training section of the Centre provides long-term care staff with the opportunity to become Certified Validation therapists. As certification becomes the norm rather than the exception, the use and practice of Validation will become more widespread.

USING VALIDATION AT THE SOUTH PORT COMMUNITY NURSING HOME IN AUSTRALIA

Alan Johns, Regional Director Eldercare, Inc, Black Forest, South Australia, and Colin Sharp, Ph.D., Associate Professor of Management, Flinders University, South Australia

In 1988, the authors conducted a study of the effectiveness of Validation using two nursing homes in Melbourne, Australia. Validation was used with 19 elderly residents at the South Port Community Nursing Home. The behavior of these residents was compared with that of 18 elderly residents at St. Anne's (Anglican) Nursing Home, whose staff did not have a formal training program in Validation Therapy. Both homes were considered to be high quality facilities, and both were willing to try innovative approaches to resident care. Indeed, some staff of both nursing homes knew about Validation. The results showed that more of the residents whose staff received Validation training improved, and fewer deteriorated over the course of the study.

Validation was introduced in Australia in the early 1980s. Although a growing number of practitioners and facilities adopted Validation and recognized its effectiveness, no research had been published in Australia investigating the effectiveness of Validation. To fill that gap, we conducted a controlled study of Validation by comparing two similar groups of elderly nursing home residents. Both of the nursing homes that participated in the study, South Port Nursing Home and St. Anne's Nursing Home, were nonprofit organizations with high standards of care. Both were located in Melbourne and some staff in both facilities knew about

Validation. Residents selected for the study in each facility were similar. The average age of South Port residents was 87.1 years; the average of St. Anne's residents was 89.7 years.

All appropriate residents in South Port were systematically given Validation therapy during the staff training program. St. Anne's staff were not formally trained, nor were residents systematically treated using Validation. Residents in both facilities were excluded from the observation and data collection of the program if they had histories or exhibited symptoms of chronic alcoholism, severe hearing impairment, severe dysphasia/dysarthria, long-term psychiatric conditions, or very poor health. In both facilities, residents whose first language was not English were excluded from the study. These criteria were established in order to minimize the number of variables influencing our results.

Three workshops and a follow-up session were held to train staff at South Port in Validation. These workshops introduced the concept of Validation, identified the types of people who benefit from Validation, described the stages of Resolution, and presented the techniques of Validation. The follow-up session, which was held 1 month after the last workshop, allowed staff to report on their progress in implementing Validation.

In order to evaluate how well Validation works, we used four measures of behavior, including the Benedictine Disorientation Checklist, Moorfield's Behavior Problem Checklist, and the Goal Attainment Scale (G.A.S.). We also used a subjective measure of change, vis-a-vis staff consensus. Using the checklists, we evaluated the behavior of the South Port residents before and 13 weeks after introducing Validation. The St. Anne's residents were also similarly assessed at the start and end of the study period.

Both the Benedictine Disorientation Checklist and Moorfield's Behavior Problem Checklist revealed significant differences between the levels of progress made by the residents in the two facilities, with South Port residents showing more progress overall. Also, South Port staff used a weekly goal attainment scale to monitor improvement of residents, which contributed to the effectiveness of Validation therapy.

Staff consensus at the two facilities indicated that almost half of the participating South Port residents (8 of 19) improved. Staff at St. Anne's reported that only 1 of the 18 participating residents improved. Of the 8 South Port residents who made substantial improvements, one example illustrates very dramatic results. This resident was virtually mute when admitted to the facility. She engaged in the repetitive motion of hand-sucking and spoke only with her hand in her mouth. Following the introduction of Validation, her hand-sucking subsided, she engaged in some meaningful conversations, and she began to relate to other residents on her ward.

Much additional research needs to be done on Validation. Our study pertained only to relatively healthy residents and these results cannot be generalized to residents who are in poor health. Our study could look only tangentially at family involvement, an important issue that warrants further study. Research on the potential role of G.A.S. in Validation therapy would clarify its benefits here. For the sample of residents we studied, however, our results suggested that Validation is effective in promoting positive changes of behavior with disoriented residents.

Francois Blanchard, Jean Prentczynski, Catherine Wong, Bernard Lamaze, Isabella Morrone, Patrick Bocquet and Damien Jolly

Hôpital Sebastopol in Reims, France, is a public university hospital. It had a 54-bed geriatric short-stay intensive care ward at the time of this writing. The unit tended to attract very old patients, about a quarter of whom showed signs of mental confusion and/or problematic behavior. The hospital sought ways of dealing with these confused patients, both to ease their anguish and to facilitate medical care.

Although Validation has been used primarily in long-term care facilities, our hope was to introduce it into the hospital in order to achieve the following goals:

1. To offer better care for our older patients suffering from psychological disorders by using alternatives to psychotropic medications

2. To reduce the tendency to hospitalize older people who lose psychological control

3. To prevent older patients from deteriorating psychologically after their hospitalization

4. To give the nursing staff a better understanding of certain behavioral disorders and to familiarize them with an alternative form of communication intervention

In trying to use Validation in an acute care hospital, we recognized that we faced major obstacles. First, the serious medical conditions of patients admitted to an intensive care unit require that medical treatment be the primary concern. Patients admitted to our unit were often very ill. Neither their poor health nor the series of tests these patients were required to undergo was conducive to building a trusting environment, in which Validation should ideally take place. Second, the average length of stay for our patients was only 10 days. This short period did not permit continuous treatment over several weeks or months, as indicated by Mrs. Feil.

Despite the obvious obstacles, we ran a pilot study on the effectiveness of Validation in our hospital. Medical and nursing staff who volunteered to participate in this study learned the basic principles of Validation by attending a 2-day seminar. They later attended a 2-day intensive workshop led by Naomi Feil. These volunteers consisted of the head of the ward, the ward psychiatrist, a member of the medical staff, and 15 nurses.

Patients at high risk for rapid deterioration were selected for the study by the ward psychiatrist. Validation caregivers were asked to meet with these patients as often as possible to establish a relationship based on trust and compassion. These 10-minute sessions were held several times a day when no other treatments were being given to the patients. Validation also was used during medical treatments and while hygienic care was being given. Volunteers from the nursing and medical staff met once a week to share their observations about each patient and to assess the changes observed.

Throughout the project, we had to face some unsolved problems:

1. Because the workload in an acute care hospital varies and medical treatment must always be the top priority,

it was not always possible to be attentive to Validation techniques. In our hospital, where participation in the project was voluntary, the problem was compounded by the fact that not all nursing staff participated in the program. This lead to complex and conflictual situations. It was impossible to ensure continuity of the Validation for each patient. Moreover, caregivers who did try to use Validation became discouraged by the fact that the high level of personal investment they made was not being made by all staff.

2. Selection of appropriate patients for Validation can be difficult in an acute care setting, because many of the people admitted suffer from severe organic diseases and some suffer from genuine dementia (i.e., Alzheimer's disease). These patients would not benefit from Validation.

3. Stopping Validation after the patient's release from the hospital was sometimes problematic. For many of our patients, the positive results of Validation were sustained after their release; others regressed, sometimes very severely (one patient died within 7 days of release).

Notwithstanding the far-from-ideal conditions in our unit, our experience with using Validation was a positive one, and we enjoyed several important changes as a result of its use:

1. Validation metamorphosized our nurses' view of disoriented older patients and taught them how to treat these patients with more compassion. As a result of Validation, the nursing and medical staff learned to understand certain kinds of behavior that previously had

troubled them. Behaviors that staff once derided were viewed with empathy. Validation gave a more human meaning to the care.

2. This attitude contributed to the diminishing of anxiety or aggressiveness and provided a more positive experience of hospitalization to patients who were already physically and psychologically fragile. Some patients even improved their ability to communicate.

3. We reduced the use of psychotropic medications on our unit. In fact, some patients who had been using such medications prior to hospitalization left the hospital free of these drugs.

4. Families and friends of these patients generally looked favorably upon Validation, and some even took an active part in the approach.

5. A better quality of life was provided for our patients during their hospitalization, and the "sliding syndrome," whereby patients deteriorate during hospitalization was often prevented. We also observed more satisfying co-operation of medical treatments and physical treatment, which helped reduce the overload of work.

6. Patients displayed less aggressiveness during hospitalization. With some, the ability to communicate improved, thereby enabling them to acknowledge and accept the final stage of their lives.

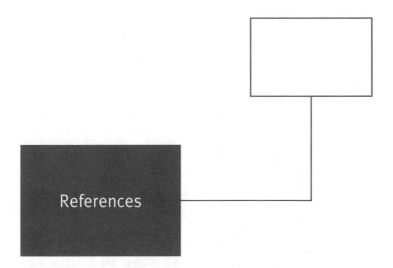

References

Alprin, S. (1980). *The study to determine the results of implementing Validation therapy.* Unpublished study. Cleveland State University, OH.

Alzheimer, A. (1907). Uber eine eigenartige Erkranjung der Hirnrinde. *Allgemeine Zeitshrift für Psychiatrie, 64,* 146–148.

Butler, R. (1963). The life review: An interpretation of reminiscence in the aged. *Psychiatry, 26,* 65–75.

Butler, R.N., & Lewis, M.I. (Eds.). (1977). *Aging and mental health.* New York: C.V. Mosby Co.

Dietch, J.T., Hewett, L.J., & Jones, S. (1989). Adverse effects of reality orientation. *Journal of the American Geriatrics Society, 37,* 974–976.

Erikson, E. (1963). *Childhood and society.* New York: Norton.

Feil, N. (1967). Group therapy in a home for the aged. *The Gerontologist, 7,* 192–195.

Feil, N. (1972). A new approach to group therapy: *The Tuesday group* (Film). Cleveland, OH: Feil Productions.

Feil, N. (1973). *A new life for Rose* (Film). Cleveland, OH: Feil Productions.

Feil, N. (1974). *Living the second time around* (Film). Cleveland, OH: Feil Productions.

Feil, N. (1978). *Looking for yesterday* (Film). Cleveland, OH: Feil Productions.

Feil, N. (1980). *The more we get together* (Film and videotape). Cleveland, OH: Feil Productions.

Feil, N. (1982). Group work with disoriented nursing home residents. *Social Work with Groups, 5*(2), 57.

Feil, N. (1985). Resolution: The final life task. *Journal of Humanistic Psychology, 25,* 91–105.

Feil, N. (1989). Validation: An empathetic approach to the care of dementia. *Clinical Gerontologist, 8,* 89–94.

Feil, N. (1991). Validation therapy. In P.K.H. Kim (Ed.), *Serving the elderly* (pp. 89–115). New York: Aldine de Gruyter.

Feil, N. (1992a). Validation therapy with late onset dementia populations. In G. Jones, & B.M.L. Miesen (Eds.), *Caregiving in dementia* (pp. 199–218). London: Routledge.

Feil, N. (1992b). *VIF Validation: The Feil method* (Rev. ed). Cleveland, OH: Feil Productions.

Feil, N. (1992c). *Sara's choice* (Videotape). Cleveland, OH: Feil Productions.

Feil, N., & Flynn, J. (1983). Meaning behind movements of the disoriented old-old. *Somatics, 4,* 4–10.

Feil, N., Shove, L., & Davenport, S. (1972). *Pilot study: A new approach for disoriented nursing home residents in a home for the aged.* Paper presented at the International Gerontological Society, Puerto Rico.

Fritz, P. (1986, November). *The language of resolution among the old-old: The effect of Validation therapy on two levels of cognitive confusion.* Paper presented at the Speech Communication Association, Chicago.

Gajdusek, D.C. (1985). Hypothesis: Interference with axonal transport of neurofilament as a common pathogenetic mechanism in certain diseases of the central nervous system. *New England Journal of Medicine, 312,* 714–719.

Jones, G. (1964, Winter). Remotivation in the aged. *Geriatric Institutions, 5*–7.

Jones, G., & Miesen, B.M.L. (Eds.). (1992). *Caregiving in dementia.* London: Routledge.

Kim, P.K.H. (Ed.). (1991). *Serving the elderly.* New York: Aldine de Gruyter.

Kral, V.A. (1977). In R.N. Butler, & M.I. Lewis (Eds.), *Aging and mental health* (pp. 76–88). New York: C.V. Mosby.

Miller, B.L. (1988). Clinical aspects of Alzheimer disease. *Annals of Internal Medicine, 109,* 41–54.

Morton, I., & Bleathman, C. (1988). Does it matter whether it's Tuesday or Friday? *Nursing Times, 84*(6), 25–27.

Neugarten, B. (1970). Dynamics of transition of middle age to old age adaptation and the life cycle. *Journal of Geriatric Psychiatry, 1*(4).

O'Connor, J., & Seymour, J. (1990). *Introducing neurolinguistic programming.* London: Hammersmith.

Peoples, M. (1982). *Validation therapy versus reality orientation as treatment for disoriented institutionalized elderly.* Unpublished master's thesis, College of Nursing, University of Akron, OH.

Prentczynski, J. (1991). *La personne agee en perte d'autonomie psychique: La methode de validation et ses apports dans un service de gerontologie.* Unpublished doctoral thesis, Department of Medicine, University of Reims, France.

Ronaldson, S., & McLaren, H. (1991). *A time to care.* Victoria, Australia: High Plains Press.

Rubin B. (1982). *Burnout: Causation and measurement.* Unpublished master's thesis, Department of Psychology, Michigan State University, East Lansing.

Selkoe, D.J. (1991, November). Amyloid protein and Alzheimer's disease. *Scientific American, 265*(5), 40–47.

Sharp, C., & Johns, A. (1991, November). *Validation therapy: An evaluation of a program at the South Port Community Nursing Home in Melbourne, Australia.* Paper presented at the Australian Association of Voluntary Care Associations, Victoria, Australia.

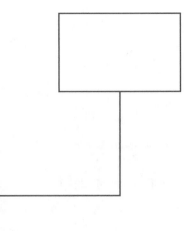

Index

Page numbers followed by t and f denote tables and figures, respectively.